"This book will be of interest to those who are approaching Bion for the first time, to those who are specifically studying Bion's *Transformations*, but also to a general psychoanalytic readership who are interested in the metapsychological and epistemological implications of the concept of transformation. I find this book particularly well calibrated towards a broad readership: the academic specialist, the well-read and mature psychoanalytic reader, and the novice. In this book, the authors apply a distinctive reading method specifically to Bion's *Transformations* (1965). It is a psychoanalytic deconstructive reading suitable to the exercise of (clinical) imagination, parameterized by consistent epistemological principles, the authors constantly focus and defocus the diverse statutes of the concept of transformations, with his vast and refined philosophical knowledge. This book will inspire many readings and re-readings of Bion, a seminal author."

Elias Mallet da Rocha Barros is a training and supervising analyst and docent at the Brazilian Psychoanalytic Society of São Paulo (SBPSP); fellow of the British Psychoanalytic Society and Institute; past editor for Latin America for the *International Journal of Psychoanalysis*; co-chair for Latin America of the IPA Encyclopedic Dictionary of Psychoanalysis; and the recipient of the 1999 Mary Sigourney Trust Award. He is also a Distinguished Fellow of the British Psychoanalytical Society.

W0234921

Reading Bion's *Transformations*

Reading Bion's Transformations is an in-depth reading of Bion's 1965 work, *Transformations*, and investigates the epistemological concept of "O" introduced by Bion.

Throughout the book, Bion's conceptual and unconventional text is discussed step-by-step, with a focus on the first three and last three chapters. The epistemological references are highlighted and analysed, allowing the reader insight into how to do a deconstructive psychoanalytic reading, acknowledging that Bion raised psychoanalytical thought and practice to new levels. The authors' reading both de-focuses and re-focuses several theoretical statutes of O discussed by Bion in 1965.

Reading Bion's Transformations is an essential read for those approaching Bion's work for the first time, as well as those seeking to better understand his theories and the metapsychological and epistemological impact of the concept of transformation within psychoanalysis.

Luís Cláudio Figueiredo, Psychoanalyst, PhD, retired Professor at the Institute of Psychology at the University of Sao Paulo – IPUSP; Professor and Research Supervisor for Master's and PhD students in the Clinical Psychology Postgraduate Program at Pontifical Catholic University of São Paulo; Member of the Psychoanalytic Circle of Rio de Janeiro; and author of 25 books on psychoanalysis in Portuguese, as well as numerous articles.

Marina F.R. Ribeiro, Psychoanalyst, PhD, Associate Professor and Research Supervisor for Master's and PhD students in the Clinical Psychology Postgraduate Program at the University of São Paulo, and author of several books and papers in both Portuguese and English, including *Why Read Ogden? The Importance of Thomas Ogden's Work for Contemporary Psychoanalysis* (Routledge, 2025).

Gina Tamburrino, Psychoanalyst, PhD, Professor and Clinical Supervisor at the Department of Training in Psychoanalysis at the Institute Sedes Sapientiae; Full Member of the Psychoanalysis Department at Institute Sedes Sapientiae; Professor and Coordinator of the course "Beyond countertransference: the implied psychoanalyst," at the same institute; and author of several books and papers.

The Routledge Wilfred R. Bion Studies Book Series

The contributions of Wilfred Bion are among the most cited in the analytic literature. Their appeal lies not only in their content and explanatory value, but in their generative potential. Although Bion's training and many of his clinical instincts were deeply rooted in the classical tradition of Melanie Klein, his ideas have a potentially universal appeal. Rather than emphasizing a particular psychic content (e.g., Oedipal conflicts in need of resolution; splits that needed to be healed; preconceived transferences that must be allowed to form and flourish, etc.), he tried to help open and prepare the mind of the analyst (without memory, desire or theoretical preconception) for the encounter with the patient.

Bion's formulations of group mentality and the psychotic and non-psychotic portions of the mind, his theory of thinking and emphasis on facing and articulating the truth of one's existence so that one might truly learn first hand from one's own experience, his description of psychic development (alpha function and container/contained) and his exploration of O are "non-denominational" concepts that defy relegation to a particular school or orientation of psychoanalysis. Consequently, his ideas have taken root in many places.... and those ideas continue to inform many different branches of psychoanalytic inquiry and interest.[1]

It is with this heritage and its promise for the future developments of psychoanalysis in mind that we present *The Routledge Wilfred Bion Studies Book Series*. This series gathers together under newly emerging and continually evolving contributions to psychoanalytic thinking that rest upon Bion's foundational texts and explore and extend the implications of his thought. For a full list of titles in the series, please visit the Routledge website at: https://www.routledge.com/The-Routledge-Wilfred-Bion-Studies-Book-Series/book-series/RWBSBS

---

1 Levine, H.B. and Civitarese, G. (2016). Editors' Preface, *The W.R. Bion Tradition*, Levine and Civitarese, eds., London: Karnac 2016, p. xxi.

Reading Bion's *Transformations*

Luís Cláudio Figueiredo, Marina F.R. Ribeiro and Gina Tamburrino

Translator: Davi Berciano Flores
Revisor: Taís de O. Nicoletti

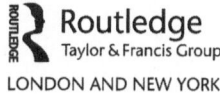

Routledge
Taylor & Francis Group

LONDON AND NEW YORK

Designed cover image: © Marina F.R. Ribeiro

First published 2025
by Routledge
4 Park Square, Milton Park, Abingdon, Oxon OX14 4RN

and by Routledge
605 Third Avenue, New York, NY 10158

Routledge is an imprint of the Taylor & Francis Group, an informa business

© 2025 Luís Cláudio Figueiredo, Marina F.R. Ribeiro, and Gina Tamburrino

British Library Cataloguing-in-Publication Data
A catalogue record for this book is available from the British Library

ISBN: 978-1-032-75998-2 (hbk)
ISBN: 978-1-032-74835-1 (pbk)
ISBN: 978-1-003-47657-3 (ebk)

DOI: 10.4324/9781003476573

Typeset in Times New Roman
by Taylor & Francis Books

Contents

Acknowledgements

True novelty is that which does not grow old with the passing of time, becoming, perhaps, even better understood. This is the case, I believe, of the reading Luís Cláudio Figueiredo made of the book *Transformations* in March 2000, with his postgraduate students at PUCSP as his interlocutors.

The moment at which those lessons took place is quite important, since very few papers referred to this shift in Bion's work during the 2000s. Particularly in regard to the statute of O, of Being and of become oneself, which are precisely examined in this reading of *Transformations*, and what has been currently discussed amongst experts in Bion's work: the clinical statute of transformations in K and O.

In 2008, Gina Tamburrino and I were following a PhD program and Luís Cláudio was our advisor. On that occasion he made available for us his notes on the 2000 classes so that we could organize a seminar on *Transformations*. We were greatly impacted by the originality and complexity of those notes, and, without any hesitation, we commented that it would be interesting to publish that material. Luís Cláudio invited us to organize and edit those precious notations and the book was published in Portuguese in 2011, with the title *Bion in Nine Lessons: Reading Transformations*.

The origin of this text lies in the seminars given by Luís Cláudio Figueiredo to his postgraduate students, hence we have kept the chapters numbered as lessons. The original title has a paradoxical, humorous character, since the book is not about introducing Bion in nine lessons, but about offering a complex reading of *Transformations* (1965). Furthermore, the title in English allows a second comprehension: that Figueiredo follows closely the vestiges left by Bion of his own transformations as a thinker of the psychoanalytic clinic and theory. Psychoanalytic thoughts seek authors in different geographic and psychic continents; the books are written in diverse languages and times; nevertheless, they can interconnect, even if only partially, in their textuality.

Thanks are due to Luís Cláudio Figueiredo, who was so generous in agreeing to publish his ideas for English-speaking readers; thanks also to my colleague Gina Tamburrino, who also supported the idea.

To Elias da Rocha Barros for the preface to this English edition, and also for his encouragement to translate and publish the book, which was fundamental.

To Howard Levine for his interest in the ideas contained in this book and for his diligent orientation towards the writing of an introduction to guide the English-speaking reader to the challenges of reading the text – both the original text by Bion, *Transformations*, as well as the readings presented in this book.

Translating is, in part, a betrayal of the original text. Portuguese and English are languages with completely different structures, which makes the venture of translation a risky and arduous task. We thank Davi B. Flores, the translator, and Taís de O. Nicoletti, the translation revisor, who accepted the challenge of translating to English an already difficult and complex book in its original language, Portuguese. They are psychoanalysts and researchers interested in Bion's work, and both take part in my research group at Universidade de São Paulo (USP) and at LipSic[1] (Interinstitutional Laboratory for Studies on Intersubjectivity and Contemporary Psychoanalysis IPUSP – PUCSP).

I thank Evelise de Souza Marra, co-organizer of the conferences on Bion's work that have taken place in São Paulo since 2008, which have been carried out with the collaboration of other colleagues from Sociedade Brasileira de Psicanálise de São Paulo (SBPSP) – Brazilian Psychoanalytic Society of São Paulo. Up to the present date there have been fifteen conferences and given the written production generated from these fruitful events (several papers and five books), they maintain Bion's legacy in Brazil in constant expansion. And now part of this consistent Brazilian output is presented to the English-speaking reader, with Howard Levine as editor.

Marina F.R. Ribeiro

Note

1   Luís Cláudio Figueiredo is currently one of LipSic's academic advisors.

Foreword

I would like to begin by briefly introducing the author of this book, Luís Cláudio Figueiredo, the professor of the seminar transcribed here, which was edited and reconstructed by Marina F.R. Ribeiro and Gina Tamburrino.

Luís Cláudio Figueiredo (henceforth Figueiredo) is a renowned and respected university professor, psychoanalyst, author of a number of scientific papers and books, and amongst the most cited psychoanalysts in Brazil. Figueiredo is a brilliant teacher in many respects. He is immensely gifted as a close reader of psychoanalytic texts, has a wonderfully clear grasp of the broad trends and movements within the conceptual and epistemological history of psychology and psychoanalysis, and is highly adept at tracing the contemporary clinical impact of ideas generated throughout the history of psychoanalysis. He adopts a way of reading texts through an interpretative and deconstructive analytic stance, followed by a reconstruction of the author or writing under examination. This twin movement of a *micro*scopic and *macro*scopic approach – deconstruction, close-examination and reconstruction – is highly useful in grasping the wider implications of the classics in psychoanalytic literature. Furthermore, he is a healthily non-sectarian reader, keen to present an author's ideas in his or her own terms without a view to "preach" or convert his readership to an author's way of thinking. At the same time, he is far from being a *naive* reader of any kind, and always incorporates a sceptical and critical view of the material under examination.

I have learnt a great deal through my reading of Figueiredo's many books. He is the co-author – alongside Elisa Ulhôa Cintra – of what I consider an absolutely splendid and original short introduction to the writings of Melanie Klein, sadly unavailable in English: *Melanie Klein: Her Style and Her Thought*[1] (2004): an exceptional guide to the thinking and the writing style of Klein, ideal for both beginners and seasoned readers. Figueiredo also co-authored, with Nelson E. Coelho Jr., another impactful book (also as yet unavailable in English), whose title could be rendered as *Psychic Ailments and Cure Strategies: Matrices and Models in Psychoanalysis* (2018),[2] which I easily count as amongst the most interesting psychoanalytic books I have recently read. In its pages, the authors postulate two large matrices (or traditions of thinking) in psychoanalysis: a Freudian-Kleinian matrix and a Ferenczian matrix. The matrices correspond to forms of ailments, and to each of them there is a corresponding cure strategy. The authors consider Bion a representative of the Freudian-Kleinian matrix, and Winnicott a representative of the Ferenczian, both being present in what they called the "transmatricial" elaborations. In the book referred to earlier, Coelho Jr. and Figueiredo (2018) propose that contemporary psychoanalysis becomes progressively *transmatricial*, that is, psychoanalysis, throughout its several flowering stages, crosses paradigms. The authors also examine contributions by André Green, Thomas Ogden, René Roussillon and Anne Alvarez, psychoanalysts they consider transmatricial. This is a very interesting take on the broad strokes of the history of psychoanalytic thought and a very interesting defence of a more embracing way forward.

Marina F.R. Ribeiro and Gina Tamburrino are Figueiredo's co-authors in the book on Bion's *Transformations* being presented here, and also in a book on Balint (2021).[3] Marina Ribeiro's style is profound and elegantly constructed at the same time; it is always a great pleasure to read what she writes. Marina is a professor at the Institute of Psychology (IP) at the prestigious University of São Paulo (USP), where she is an advisor in masters and PhD programs. Furthermore, she is the author of the books *From Mother into Daughter: Transmission of Femininity* (2011) and *Infertility and Assisted Reproduction: Wishing to Have Children in Contemporary Families* (2004). She is co-author, with Elisa Ulhôa Cintra, of the book *Why Klein?* (2018), organizer and author of the books *Beyond Countertransference: The Implicated Psychoanalyst* (2017) and *Melanie Klein in Contemporary Psychoanalysis: Theory, Clinic and Culture* (2019).

Gina Tamburrino is a psychoanalyst, professor, and clinical supervisor at the Department of Psychoanalysis at the Institute *Sedes Sapientiae*. She is a full Member of the Department of Psychoanalysis and author of the books *Listening through Images* (2007) and *Enactments and Transformations in the Analytic Field* (2016).

The present book will be of interest to those who are approaching Bion for the first time, to those who are specifically studying Bion's *Transformations*, but also to a general psychoanalytic readership who are interested in the metapsychological and epistemological implications of the concept of transformation. It is a book which I find particularly well calibrated both towards a broad readership: the academic specialist, the well-read and mature psychoanalytic reader, and the novate.

In this book Figueiredo applies his distinctive reading method specifically to Bion's *Transformations* (1965). It is a psychoanalytic deconstructive reading suitable to the exercise of (clinical) imagination, parameterized by consistent epistemological principles. As Marina writes in the introduction, Figueiredo constantly focuses and defocuses the diverse statutes of the concept of transformations, with his vast and refined philosophical knowledge.

What pleases me the most when reading these seminars is the feeling of the absence of idealization and partisanship of the one conducting it (Figueiredo), and of those who edited them (Ribeiro and Tamburrino). They invite their readers to build together ever-changing hypotheses on the meaning of what is being addressed, without idealizing the psychoanalytic author (in this case, Bion), nor attempting to "win the reader over" to a specific and preconceived position.

The classes presented in this book are a guide through Bion's entire book, *Transformations*, emphasizing the transformations that operate on the text itself, from the point of view of its impact and meaning, which also constitutes the movement that Octavio Paz (1984) called intertextuality: that texts from the different times – present, past, and future – interact amongst themselves, producing new meanings and erasing others.

This book, supplemented with Marina's introduction for the English edition, is original for being dedicated to investigating the epistemological statutes of the concept of 'O', or, to put it more accurately, of the hypothesis of 'O' as something potentially useful for us to understand the evolution (or maturation) of the psyche, or even the possibility of its involution.

Transformation is not a synonym to psychic change, although it comprises this dimension. It is a larger entity, more mysterious, for it remains an open concept (Eco [1962] 1989)[4] bearing large philosophical implications on the intimate character of Being, be it strictly from a psychoanalytic point of view or from a point of view of Being as a metaphysical concept or entity.

In the introduction to this book, Marina, while following closely Bion's text ([1970] 2014), affirms something that deserves deeper scrutiny: she states that the analyst cannot be *identified* with O, but must *be* it. This is somewhat a recursive proposition, as the concept itself is used to construct the affirmation. This idea has metaphysical and clinical implications: it says something about the very nature of Being. The book proposes that the transformations in O occur out of the representational domain, an unsettling affirmation which produces consequences to the theory of the constitution of the psyche as much as to the psychoanalytic clinic.

In this context, Marina addresses Luís Cláudio's reading of Bion's text as something similar to the psychoanalytic interpretation in the session: something beyond intellectual comprehension. The patient, as well as the reader or the students in these seminars, are modified by the text, the act of reading turns into a transforming and transformative experience. It is a curious experience as far as it cannot be explained nor understood immediately, it must be matured, "cured" in the sense of the "curing" of meat and cheeses that undergo complex changes on the way to improvement and an acquisition of nuances in flavours and textures. When this experience becomes thinkable it gains existence as something alive, in constant change. It is in this sense that the transformation in O goes beyond what we usually call psychic change. Its effect is hard to describe and parametrize.

It is clear in these seminars that the transformation in O itself, that which leads the patient to meet the *himself/self*, is subject to the movement of O itself. The *oneself* is a transitional state, a *coming into being* subjacent to the *becoming*.

Bion, as Luís Cláudio, Marina and Gina say, when working with the concept of *becoming O in its relation to K and vice-versa*, is inspired by Nietzsche. Probably, when Nietzsche thinks of life as literature (Nehamas, 1985), it is in the sense that a knowledge (K) can transform the life of a character in a fiction written by himself, so that in the following instant, he becomes a non-fictional, real being for then becoming a character again, and so it goes endlessly. To know (K) comprises two movements: one is of cognitive/intellectual nature, the other is an intuitive capturing, being of an epiphany's nature. Nehamas (1985, p. 189) writes:[5]

> More important, however, is the fact that so long we are alive, we are always finding ourselves in new and unforeseen situations; we constantly have new thoughts and desires, we continue to perform new actions. In their light we may at any point come to face the need to reinterpret, to reorganize, or even to abandon early ones.

This point becomes clearer when Figueiredo describes the third possibility of *becoming O* as being similar to the Kantian *thing in itself* and, following that, cites Bion to illustrate, after mentioning a passage from the poem *Paradise Lost* by Milton. Let's look at Milton's verses and Bion's comments on them:

> The rising world of waters dark and deep
> Won from the void and formless infinite

Bion ([1965] 2014, p. 262) comments:

> I am not interpreting what Milton says but using it to represent O. The process of binding is a part of the procedure by which something is "won from the void and formless infinite"; it is K and must be distinguished from the process by which O is 'become'. The sense of inside and outside, internal and external objects.

This matter evokes a passage, not mentioned by the authors, which is present in *Cogitations*. In that book, Bion exemplifies his conception of dream work alpha through a situation in which he imagines himself answering to a friend who has asked him where he plans to spend his holidays, Bion writes:

> ... suppose I am talking to a friend who asks me where I propose to spend my holiday; as he does so, I visualize the church of a small town not far from the village in which I propose to stay. The small town is

important because it possesses the railway station nearest to my village. Before he has finished speaking, a new image has formed, and so on.

The image of the church has been established on a previous occasion – I cannot now tell when. Its evocation in the situation I am describing would surprise no one, but what I now wish to add may be more controversial. I suggest that the experience of this particular conversation with my friend and this particular moment of the conversation – not simply his words but the totality of that moment of experience – is being perceived sensorially by me and converted into an image of that particular village church.

I do not know what else may be going on, though I am sure that much more takes place than I am aware of. But the transformation of my sense impressions into this visual image is part of a process of mental assimilation. The impressions of the event are being re-shaped as a visual image of that particular church, and so are being made into a form suitable for storage in my mind.

(Bion [1992] 2014, p. 174, our emphasis)

It is this process of mental assimilation, of non-sensorial nature, which comes from the totality of the experience's moment, that becomes the base of an intuitive emotional experience, via evocation.

Bion makes use of this example to entertain the possibility that a similar process might take place between analyst and patient in a session. Moreover, that certain patients might be unable to transform the images of sensorial impressions that arise in the session into forms suitable for mental storage.

The evocation of the church illustrates the idea of the existence of a void and formless infinite from which the experience emerges. It is important to note that the church's image is not reduced to a memory, but it is, above all, a figuration that evokes an experience, producing something that emerges, as in a fiction, when a character comes up, makes a solid and deep impact, and then disappears. Marina, in her introduction to this book, presents a similar clinical vignette: she describes her evocation of the shoes of a dead man when meeting a patient for the first time. Both Figueiredo and Marina are describing the process through which the evolution of the symbolic forms operates, ideas that I find are close some musings of my own, which were developed in texts I have already published together with Elizabeth da Rocha Barros (2011, 2016).[6]

I shall conclude by saying that this book will inspire many readings and re-readings of Bion, a seminal author.

Elias Mallet da Rocha Barros[7]
São Paulo, March 2021

Notes

1 T.N.: The title may be loosely translated as "Melanie Klein: Style and Thinking".
2 T.N.: The title may be loosely translated as "Psychic Ailments and Cure Strategies: Matrices and Models in Psychoanalysis".
3 T.N.: The title may be loosely translated as "Balint in Seven Lessons".
4 Umberto Eco ([1962] 1989) *The Open Work* (Cambridge, MA: Harvard University Press).
5 A. Nehamas (1985) *Nietzsche Life as Literature* (Cambridge, MA and London: Harvard University Press).
6 E.M. da Rocha Barros and E.L. da Rocha Barros (2011) Reflections on the Clinical Implications of Symbols. *International Journal of Psychoanalysis*, 92(4): 879–901; E. M. da Rocha Barros and E.L. da Rocha Barros (2016) The Function of Evocation in the Working Through of the Countertransference: Projective Identification, Reverie and the Expressive Function of the Mind-Reflection Inspired by Bion's Work, In: H. Levine and G. Civitarese (2016) (eds), *The W.R. Bion Tradition* (London: Routledge), pp. 141–154.
7 Elias Mallet da Rocha Barros is a training and supervising analyst and docent at the Brazilian Psychoanalytic Society of São Paulo (SBPSP); Fellow of the British Psychoanalytic Society and Institute; past editor for Latin America for the *International Journal of Psychoanalysis*; co-chair for Latin America of the *IPA Encyclopedic Dictionary of Psychoanalysis* and the recipient of the 1999 Mary Sigourney Trust Award. He is also a Distinguished Fellow of the British Psychoanalytical Society.

References

Bion, W.R. ([1965] 2014). Transformations. In: *The Complete Works of W.R. Bion, Vol. V*, ed. C. Mawson. London: Karnac Books, pp. 115–280.
Bion, W.R. ([1970] 2014). Attention and Interpretation: A Scientific Approach to Insight in Psycho-Analysis and Groups. In: *The Complete Works of W.R. Bion, Vol. VI*, ed. C. Mawson. London: Karnac Books.
Bion, W.R. ([1992] 2014). Cogitations. In: *The Complete Works of W.R. Bion, Vol. XI*, ed. C. Mawson. London: Karnac Books, pp. 1–350.
Eco, U. (1989). *The Open Work*. Cambridge, MA: Harvard University Press.
Nehamas, A. (1985). *Nietzsche: Life as Literature*. Cambridge, MA and London: Harvard University Press.
Rocha Barros, E.M. da and E.L. da Rocha Barros (2011). Reflections on the Clinical Implications of Symbols. *International Journal of Psychoanalysis*, 92(4): 879–901.
Rocha Barros, E.M. da and E.L. da Rocha Barros (2016). The Function of Evocation in the Working Through of the Countertransference: Projective Identification, Reverie and the Expressive Function of the Mind-Reflection Inspired by Bion's Work. In: H. Levine and G. Civitarese (eds), *The W.R. Bion Tradition*. London: Routledge, pp. 141–154.

Introduction to the English edition

This introduction intends to emphasize the importance of studying *Transformations* (1965), the book for those who wish to deepen their understanding of Bion's work and, specifically, the change that takes place in the final chapters of *Transformations*, in which Bion moves his interest from apprehending the psychic reality, transformations in K (knowledge) to the Being, to becoming oneself, to the transformations in O.

> The analyst must focus his attention on O, the unknown and unknowable. The success of psychoanalysis depends on the maintenance of a psychoanalytic point of view; the point of view is the psychoanalytic vertex; the psychoanalytic vertex is O. With this the analyst cannot be identified: he must be it.
>
> (Bion [1970] 2014, p. 243)

To begin with,[1] *Transformations* is considered one of the most enigmatic and difficult of Bion's texts. Furthermore, the book itself can be read as the testimony of a transformation in O process; a catastrophic change, a caesura in Bion's life and work, and this introduction takes this assumption, as do other authors.

This book,[2] presented here in its English edition, aims to emphasize the importance of studying this text for those who wish to deepen their understanding of Bion's work, specifically the change that takes place in the last chapters of *Transformations*, in which Bion moves his interest from apprehending the psychic reality, transformations in K (knowledge) to the Being, to becoming oneself, to the transformations in O. The book's subtitle precisely addresses this modification: the change from learning to growth.

Transformations represents a shift in the direction Bion had been following in previous works. Before, Bion had been interested in learning from emotional experiences, that is to say, the transformations in K (knowledge), which belong to the field of representations. Upon finishing this publication, Bion dedicated himself to the transformations in O, which occur in a non-representational level of experience: in Being and in becoming oneself.

DOI: 10.4324/9781003476573-1

I find it productive and creative when a concept, in this case, caesura,[3] is used to think about the work of its own creator. The caesura occurs in *Transformations*, especially in its three last chapters. We might think of Luís Cláudio Figueiredo's[4] reading as a kind of microscopic view of this caesura – from this point of view, it is a quite unique text, even considering the vast number of publications of books and articles about Bion to this date, in both English and Portuguese.

Psychoanalysts interested in Bion's works cannot avoid dedicating themselves to the study of the ideas developed in *Transformations*. For those who are new to his works, this book may serve as a good companion to a reading of Bion's original text. And, for those who already know his works in depth, the book raises important and current epistemological questions, referring, especially, to the many O statutes which are presented by Bion in the final part of *Transformations* and highlighted by Luís Cláudio's thorough and deconstructive reading.

From Bion's insight at the end of *Transformations*, the moment at which he postulates the transformations in O, there is a catastrophic change in both his life and works. To the surprise of his British colleagues, in 1968, Bion, at the age of 71, moved to Los Angeles, California. Was this perhaps a change that reveals his commitment to his own emotional truth? A transformation in O? Figueiredo goes on to follow, in his reading, the vestiges left in the text by Bion's own transformations as a great thinker of psychoanalytic theory and practice.

During the Californian years, a creative and productive period of his life, Bion travelled four times to Brazil (in 1973, 1974, 1975 and 1978), in response to invitations from his friend and colleague Frank Philips, to give lectures, seminars and supervisions, disseminating a legacy which has generated several publications in Portuguese.

Reading Bion's Transformations is an in-depth reading of *Transformations*, a conceptual and unconventional analysis which was presented originally as graduate lectures in the early 2000s.[5] Bion's text is discussed step by step and the epistemological references are highlighted and analysed. The book addresses the first three and last three chapters of *Transformations*. The intention is to examine the capacity for a deconstructive psychoanalytic reading, acknowledging that Bion elevated psychoanalytical thought and practice to new levels.

Figueiredo's (2000, 2011) reading is constantly de-focusing and re-focusing on the several statutes of O. In sum, the main objective of *Reading Bion's Transformations* is to investigate the epistemological statutes of O in the book *Transformations* (1965); Figueiredo highlighted and problematized three of them, which will be briefly presented in this introduction.

Figueiredo (1999), finding support in Jacques Derrida postulations, demonstrates that a deconstructive reading starts by cultivating a relationship of proximity, loyalty and freedom to the text in all its dimensions. A close and deconstructive reading favours the text and the intertextuality rather than the work and its author. Even if an initial reading of a text demands a systematic approach, and also expects the text to be treated as an author's work, later, readers will need to apply themselves to a close and deconstructive reading which considers not only the text but the intertextual dialogues contained within it.

This reading method assumes that there is always an inter-textuality in each text. An author's text will refer to other texts of their own or refer to texts of other authors who came before or after; and refers us to texts that are still to be written. Bion (1965) proposes, at the beginning of *Transformations*, that this book would dismiss other books, an idea which obviously could not be sustained. *Attention and Interpretation* (1970) is an expansion of the insights of *Transformations*, especially regarding what refers to O. From the postulations on transformation in O, the psychoanalytic vertex becomes O, and no longer K. As mentioned in the opening epigraph to this introduction: the analyst cannot not be identified with O, it must be it (Bion [1970] 2014).

This promoted a shift in the comprehension of the concepts postulated by Bion before 1965, and most of all, a return – in new levels – to what Freud had proposed as the psychoanalytic method of the free-floating attention. Bion proposes that the analyst must have the discipline, when being with his analysand, to be in a state of no memory (past), no desire (future) and with no previous comprehension ([1965] 2014, [1967] 2014). The analyst must be open to the new experience which will evolve upon the meeting between the two personalities, the analyst's, and the patient's; therefore, to be adrift, and be prepared to let himself float through experiences not yet lived by the dyad. This methodological proposal is, according to Gerber and Figueiredo (2018, p. 81) a "… true renovation of the listening in free-floating attention in its ethical dimension: to listen to the other without prejudices, without filters, with no memories, no expectations or specific desires …".

Bion's work emphatically considers the complexity of the mental functioning. Moreover, it constantly sends the reader into the unknown, retaining the unsaturated text, leaving it open to other potential meanings which are always transitory. The moment we have the impression that we have understood something in our reading, we have already lost that ephemeral feeling of apprehending the content. As a result, we suggest a reading within the mental state that Bion ([1965] 2014, [1967] 2014) proposed: without memory, without desire, and without a previous comprehension – which we know to be a considerable challenge for the analyst, and even more so to some readers of psychoanalytic texts who are searching for saturated and conclusive understandings.

Grotstein (2019, p. 239) proposes a technique when reading Bion:

He later made the statement that the analyst, while listening to the patient, should really listen to himself listening to the patient. This novel 'technique' can also be applied to reading his published work, and I have every reason to believe that that was how Bion desired for readers to approach his works: to listen to their own spontaneous thoughts while reading him, i.e., their own transformations of their own personal experiences upon reading him.

Reading the text may become a transformational experience, which demands what Bion ([1970] 2014) called patience: tolerating not-knowing, being adrift. Also, having faith – which Bion denominates a scientific attitude. To have faith that some meaning will emerge from the chaos of the paranoid-schizoid state of mind, enabling one to enter in a state of safety, the depressive state of mind, thus reaching a K (knowledge), which is always provisional and transitory. Let us remember that Bion provided Kleinian concepts with significant tridimensionality, complexity, and plasticity; especially the concepts of paranoid-schizoid and depressive positions, projective identification, and envy (Cintra and Ribeiro, 2018).

There is a specificity in Luís Cláudio Figueiredo's reading of *Transformations* (1999). As previously mentioned, it is a close and deconstructive reading, sensitive to impurities, irregularities, to fractures, to the otherness of and within the text, with no idealization or partisanship, considering the complexity of the Bionian text. From this point of view, this book is also a testimony to the creative use of the deconstructive psychoanalytic reading method, besides being a study carried out at university graduate level; thus, it is a method currently used in psychoanalytic research; a sophisticated method of investigation and study of a psychoanalytic text. Bion's work is still lacking presence in university studies, therefore I believe it is crucial to introduce some of his ideas to undergraduate programs as well as postgraduate programs. I believe that the experience of openness and interest of a new generation to such an innovative author as Bion during undergraduate studies will encourage the expansion of his thought throughout future generations.

The theory of transformations is a theory of the clinical observation in the here and now of the analytical session. It is an observation of how the clinical phenomena between analyst and analysand evolve, the sequence of transformations that occurs in a session, in the analytic pair in complex interaction. It is also an observation of the interpretation, the analyst's construction, or her verbal formulation, which is understood as a product of these countless transformations occurring during an analytic session – given that the interpretation generates new transformations.

Transformations approaches the psychoanalytic efficacy, not only the truths of psychoanalytic knowledge. Bion returns to the matter of the purpose of interpretation in psychoanalysis: "If I am right in suggesting that phenomena are known but reality is 'become', the interpretation must do more than increase knowledge" (Bion [1965] 2014, p. 259). In other words, interpretation should favour a transformation in O, should favour the becoming of oneself, not only the gaining of self-knowledge.

In every transformation there is an invariance,[6] something that remains unaltered. Zimerman (2014) clarifies the concept using the example of water: as a liquid, as vaporized or as frozen, the invariant element is the H_2O molecule. Another analogy we can employ to understand this dyad of transformation/invariance is with a photograph: of a person at five years old and then at fifty years old – what is the invariance which allows an acknowledgement that it is the same person? What about the clinical material, how can we acknowledge an invariance? We understand that the invariance may favour the appearance of the selected fact – in other words, that which will be object of the analyst's interpretation, or as a fact which is fundamental for the understanding of the analysand's psychic functioning. For example: the patient's psychic suffering may be condensed into an image that emerges in the session through the analyst's capacity for reverie, as we will see in the clinical vignette presented at the end of this introduction.

Based the model presented by Bion ([1965] 2014), in which the analyst observes the reflection of trees on the lake but does not see the trees themselves, there are different degrees of distortions in what is perceived, depending on the turbulence of the water and climate conditions. The trees by the lake are a manifestation of O, for O is unknowable. The turbulence of the water and the climate conditions are the emotions that circulate in the session, in the analytic field, the L, H and K links. Bion calls these distortions hyperbolas, carrying different degrees of transformation of the original emotional experience, in the sense of a detachment, just like the ripples that move away when we throw a rock in a lake.

The transformations theory comprises and contains the Freudian theory of transference (transformations in rigid motion) and the Kleinian theory of projective identification (projective transformations). The transformation in rigid motion holds similarities with the transference as postulated by Freud, something from the patient's past is transferred to the analyst, and, in general, this is identified as an invariant, something that remains and is continuously re-introduced in the transference. In transformations in rigid motion the invariance is acknowledged quite easily.

There are the projective transformations, postulated upon the expansion of Melanie Klein's concept of projective identification. In *Learning from Experience* (1962), Bion proposed the concepts of container and contained and considered that minds communicate via projective identification, setting the Kleinian concept to a higher level of complexity, and in the intersubjective field. Projective transformations allow different degrees of distortion, the transformations in hallucinosis being the extreme limit, that is to say, the high point of hyperbolic distortion, the frontier between the mental and non-mental, in which it becomes difficult to acknowledge an invariant, given the brutal distortion.[7]

There are the transformations in K (knowledge), and, by the end of *Transformations*, Bion approached the transformations in O, the becoming oneself. The many types of transformations are oscillating vertexes, and they may occur in different moments of a session. The analysis should favour trans-formations in K and in O, the learning from experience (K) and becoming (O).[8]

From *Transformations* onward, Bion understands that contact with psychic reality occurs in a non-sensuous way, an apprehension that happens through intuition and not through sensuous intake. The being in O of the analyst, as Bion (1970) writes, is the state of mind which favours the psychoanalytic intuition when they are in contact with the patient's psychic reality, a knowledge without mediation of sensory elements. Bion ([1965] 1967) understands that memory and desire derive from the sensuous and are intensified by it, and therefore do not favour intuition, and it is for this reason that he suggests this difficult technique: analysts must attend to their patients in a mental state bearing no desire, no memory, and no previous comprehension, as if it were the first time.

In Bion's first presentation of his ideas on memory and desire, which were given at the scientific meetings of the British Society in 1965 (then published later in 1967), he says:

> Nevertheless, as analysts we do know – and I think it is borne in on us more and more as experience builds up – that we really do deal with *something*; that the psychoanalytic experience, however sceptical we may be, is really an emotional experience and it really exists, even if we shall never know or be in a position to give even an approximately correct description of what takes place. For this reason, I think – and find it most useful to do so – of any clinical description as being by nature of a pic-torial representation, or, shall we say, a sensuous representation (because I am thinking of what takes place in an analytic situation). I transform that situation into visual images and then a further transformation into verbal formulations, such as those with which we are familiar here.
>
> (Bion [1965] 2014, p. 10)

The analyst faces the challenge of dealing with that which precedes the sen-suous, the non-sensuous, captured by the psychoanalytic intuition, the mind's third eye, the way through which an unconscious captures another uncon-scious. Furthermore, analysts must deal with the sensuous, that which could be transformed in a pictorial representation by their own capacity for reverie. In addition, psychoanalysts must face the sophisticated, plastic and aesthetic capacity of transforming images emerging from the analytic encounter into words, the verbal formulations. There is also the generation of images upon interpretations or constructions made by the analyst, in a circularity that feeds back and favours psychic intimacy and the expansion of the analytic field. This is how I understand what Bion ([1965] 2014) writes regarding the diameter generated by the interpretation, which must be neither limited nor too vast, but one which favours intimate contact between two minds: the analyst's and the analysand's, in the constant transformations of an O common to the dyad.

That which may be pictured from the psychoanalytic intuition occurs beyond and before any sensuous form, or of infra and supra sensuous form (Bion [1992] 2014). Anxieties do not smell, are not visible, cannot be touched, they are intuited by the analyst's mind, says Bion ([1965] 1967). We need a beam of intense darkness to intuit in the here and now of the session, to make the invisible of the experience visible.

> Freud, in a letter to Lou Andreas-Salomé, suggested his method of achieving a state of mind which would give advantages that would compensate for obscurity when the object investigated was peculiarly obscure. He speaks of blinding himself artificially. As a method of achieving this artificial blinding I have indicated the importance of eschewing memory and desire.
>
> (Bion [1970] 2014, p. 257)

The analyst's function in the session, according to the postulation of the transformations in O, becomes a continuous oscillation between knowledge (K) and being (O). In other words, it is a continuous transformation from O to K, and from K to O, upon the crossing of hyperbolic turbulence, the always present psychic reality distortions:

> ... Bion tells us about the experience in O – the emotional experience in its Origin condition of all our somatopsychic life: it is not about 'knowing', but 'becoming', to deeply reconcile with one's own unconscious emotional experience, bare of defences and sophistry, and also without reducing this experience to the field of the senses which are vested and acknowledgeable by the consciousness. In this context, which transcends the classical epistemology since what is at stake is the correspondence between the representation and its object, occurs 'another truth', the truth in O, of major importance for the psychoanalytic clinic, whose goals are not reduced to knowing, or knowing oneself – although it involves this – but to project themselves towards an effective subjective transformation, which only happens when there is a profound and undisguised contact of the subject with himself, with the infinite unconscious that inhabits and drives him.
>
> (Figueiredo, 2014, p. 127)

Although we might think of transformations in K and in O as oscillating vertexes, the *princeps* transformation is to become: "Their value therapeutically is greater if they are conducive to transformations in O; less if conducive to transformations in K" (Bion [1970] 2014, p. 242). Bion, inspired by Nietzsche, says that in analysis the patient becomes who he is, the best he can be with what he is at each moment, since the unconscious in infinite; this is what drives us, a constant immanence.

Approaching the transformations in O, Figueiredo (2000, 2011) identifies three conceptions of O that emerge in *Transformations*. What is the conception or the statute of O in the theory scheme of *Transformations*? How does this conception oscillate throughout Bion's book?

First, there is the O evoked through platonic forms; O is inaccessible to the senses and, in itself, it does not "phenomenalize",[9] but contains the matrices of possible phenomena, that is to say, it bears an order: transcendental forms. This conception of O as platonic forms correspond to the comprehension of innate preconception, the mind's framework, the inherited trends to organize the world according to a few patterns Figueiredo (2000, 2011).

In the second conception, O does not contain the platonic forms, but a potentiality for distinctions not yet developed. Nevertheless, according to Figueiredo (2000, 2011), in this conception, the reason why resistance[10] is sparked is not understandable. What could generate resistance? When there is a movement towards O, towards the experience of the analysand's emotional truth, what could generate resistance? Bion writes that the emotional truth is what feeds the mind, but we still fear coming into contact with this truth, thus, we resist it, we resist the unknown in ourselves.

In the third, latest and utmost meaning of O as the void and formless infinite from which the world emerges still in a chaotic state, the reasons behind the emergence of resistance become understandable. Resistance is generated when facing anxiety from the void and formless infinite, that is, facing the unknown. Bion ([1965] 2014, p. 261) uses a verse by John Milton in *Paradise Lost* to represent O: "The rising world of waters dark and deep / Won from the void and formless infinite".

Figueiredo (2000, 2011) considers that it is only in this third comprehension that O corresponds to the Kantian thing in itself, which cannot be known, nevertheless its primary and secondary qualities can be apprehended. Citing Bion:

> I am not interpreting what Milton says but using it to represent O. The process of binding is a part of the procedure by which something is "won from the void and formless infinite"; it is K and must be distinguished from the process by which O is 'become'. The sense of inside and outside, internal and external objects, introjection and projection, container and contained, all are associated with K.
>
> (Bion [1965] 2014, p. 262)

As Figueiredo (2000, 2011) sees it, Bion intensifies the hiatus between the universe of concepts' logic (K) – the inside and outside sense, internal and external objects, introjection and projection, container and content – and the void and formless infinite plane on which the experience emerges. This hiatus has a significant reverberation in the theoretical universe of psychoanalysis:

the interval between knowing psychoanalysis and being psychoanalyzed, between knowing oneself and becoming oneself.

Continuing in the direction of highlighting some specific articulations present in this book to conduct and instigate a future reader, we emphasize that it is from *Transformations* (1965) onwards that the quality of transformations accomplished in the consulting room, to the analytic pair, within the analytic field, becomes crucial. To transform is to trans + form, to form beyond, which implies formative movements as much as disintegrative ones; to transform forms as much as destroy them. In the unconscious experience implied by psychoanalysis it is necessary to acknowledge the becoming dimension as much as that which is being undone, the latter being rarely highlighted in other texts. The movement of de-forming, being undone in O, is an emphasis in Figueiredo's reading (2000, 2011):

> Being become by O seems to imply a 'constructive' movement in which O imposes itself with its 'development' potential. Becoming O, understood now as a void and formless infinite, is, on the contrary, a deconstructive movement back to baseless, to the dark nights of the soul. In the first case it is *letting oneself be done by O*, in the other is *letting oneself be undone in O*.

Going in the same direction of de-forming is the book's approach and discussion on the α function and α transformation (Tα), establishing relationship between the two. It considers that Tα encompasses the α function, but is not reduced to it, since some results of transformations – given destructiveness and disintegration – cannot be considered thoughts, but evacuations and projections. The transformation is implied in forming but also in deforming, that is to say, not only thoughts might be destroyed, but also the capacity to think.

Another comprehension worth highlighting in the text presented here refers to the beta dimension of clinical material, which is always present. In Bion, the term β element and T β (β transformation), provides some confusion for the reader, as T β is a product of a transformation, and the β element is an experience in the raw stage.

The term transformation unfolds into three: Transformations (T) encompass the transformations as the process (T α) and transformations as products (T β). When we are facing T patient β, we are facing the product of a transformation: this is the clinical material that will be presented to the analyst; nevertheless, this material still contains a beta dimension. We are always looking at an infinite sequence of transformations in which the origin (O) is unknowable, and that which is presented as form, or representation remains continuously as a beta, enigmatic dimension. Bion describes the limits of representations, the constant forming and deforming, always partial, that is, the experience's beta dimension is always present. "A careful reading of Bion, however, allows us to see that it is an epistemological idea relating to the limits of representation" (Mawson 2014, p. 215).

Figueiredo (2000, 2011) would argue that the clinical material – despite already containing a few forms and patterns from which it is possible to extract invariants – is far from having the hermeticism and the univocity capable of determining once and for all the most appropriate psychoanalytic transformation, and the interpretation to be formulated. The clinical material contains an enigmatic, intrusive, disturbing beta dimension that summons the analyst to an experience that always involves emotional turbulence, a bad job, as Bion ([1979] 2014) puts it.

Could the analyst foster a transformation in O from an interpretation and from analytic knowledge? O is inaccessible to the senses and, in itself, does not 'phenomenalize' itself. However, it would already contain the matrices of the possible phenomena in itself. The experience that Bion calls mystic will be a model for this type of transformation, which is no longer a transformation *of* O, but a transformation *in* O; it is no longer a knowledge of O, but a becoming O, that is, the gap, or hiatus as Bion writes, between knowing psychoanalysis and being psychoanalyzed, between having a knowledge of oneself and becoming oneself, as previously mentioned (Bion [1970] 2014).

Although Bion does not present himself as a mystic, we are still touched by the memory that for him, searching for a suitable means of expression is necessary, even if it fails as it is always an approximation bearing distortions, writes Figueiredo (2000, 2011). Just like the mystic, the psychoanalyst has an experience of O which cannot be disqualified nor transformed in suitable representation, for every transformation of O is somehow hyperbolic. One might say that L, H and K are always unsuitable to O, although they are suitable for transformations OF O. In each of these links there is some type of exaggeration and distancing, which are in the roots of what Bion calls hyperbole.

For Bion, to be O or become O is neither a theoretical possibility nor can it be a categorical imperative, that is, superegoic, says Figueiredo (2000, 2011). This book postulates that what is present in situations of resistance is the passage to O, more than the knowledge of O. In the act of dissolving oneself in the unknown, in deep, turbid waters, resistance arises. Accepting and embracing O upon its imminence can be the best, yet painful, solution – which breaks resistance to O. Knowledge (K) can actually be one of the ways in which the transformation *in* O does not occur, a way to prevent its imminence. What is at stake is not knowledge and its vicissitudes, in other words, the cognitive capacities of men and its limits, but the terrifying possibility of passing to O, of transforming oneself in O, in its imminence and immanence: the void and formless infinite.

According to Figueiredo (2000, 2011) a pathological situation is installed when the encounter with O must be prevented and delayed infinitely. In this avoidance we only tamper with the transformations of O. That means that not only the H link prevails, but, also, when L and K prevail – situations in which O is only hyperbolically present – there is always a resistance to O operating, a resistance to the unknown.

What generates resistance is the anxiety of facing the void and formless infinite – no entities – and, probably, the terror from the world emerging from turbid and deep waters, for the world here is not conquered from nothing, in the form of something simple and well discriminated. In this version, the statue of O as unknowable finds its utmost formulation. The idea of O as the void and formless infinite – an absence of entities, in Heideggerian terms, in other words, a moment in which the world emerges in a still chaotic state. In this case it is much easier to identify the reasons behind the resistance, behind the avoidance to the unknown.

Therefore, we may suppose that O is a field of possibilities to 'evolve', which is inaccessible in itself, but whose 'products' can be known; or that O is the void and formless infinite from which one earns the secondary and primary qualities that compose the entities.

After this theoretical explanation on transformations, I will introduce a clinical vignette as a reference for us to think over the concepts. Considering that it is always challenging to articulate the clinical material with theoretical abstractions, we shall trust the encouragement and curiosity triggered by the experience:

> When I meet Antônio for the first time, having no information about him, I find myself fixated by his shoes, and I think: these are the shoes of a dead person, how can somebody wear a dead man's shoes? I realize I am having a near-hallucinatory experience, the shoes produce the effect of a magnetic field from which I cannot deviate my eyes and thoughts: I see death and I am paralyzed. He starts talking, I feel divided, observing what is being said and the intense feeling of death in which I am submerged, not understanding a thing about what is happening. I am being dragged by the disturbing experience, and I wait in a receptive silence. At the end of our encounter, Antônio tells me, in a brief and detached form, the facts of his life that still needed to be dreamt, facts that were contained and condensed in the image of the dead man shoes, a pictorial representation through which I was suddenly abducted when I met him. His only daughter had been born with several malformations, she underwent surgical interventions and lived only a few years. Antônio had come to consult with me approximately one year after the girl's death, or of his near psychic death. He walked in the shoes of a dead man, devitalized, a deceased man who was still alive. The manifested demand from his analysis was expressed through other matters: he could not find professional or financial recognition. Life was of unmatched brutality, and there he was, a man walking with death tied to his feet. And, in the same room, there was an analyst trying to dream the brutality of the facts of his life.

Returning to Bion, the origin of any transformation is unknowable, is O equally shared, even if in a diverse form, by patient and analyst in the session: "I therefore postulate that O in any analytic situation is available for transformation by analyst and analysand equally" (Bion [1965] 2014, p. 169).

The turbulence generated by meeting Antônio – the encounter of two personalities is always a bad job, as says Bion (1979) – quickly evolves through a pictorial representation, a reverie in the mind of the analyst: the image of the dead man shoes, which also becomes a selected fact of the session.

The pictorial image is already the product (T analyst β) of a transformation process (T analyst α). The analyst, in her negative capacity state (no memory, no desire, no preconceived comprehension), a mind state receptive to O, and, also, which favours the analytic intuition, is dragged by the emotional experience, momentarily senseless, staying adrift. It takes patience (paranoid-schizoid state of mind) and faith, the act of faith (Bion, 1970) that a meaning will emerge in the posteriority of the situation, generating a safe state (depressive state of mind), allowing an evolution in K, a knowledge of the patient's psychic suffering.

The experience of "seeing" the shoes of a dead man refers to what Bion ([1970] 2014, Vol. VI, p. 250) called transformation in hallucinosis:

> … to appreciate hallucination the analyst must participate in the state of hallucinosis. From what I have said it will be clear that this is so, for I have postulated that a K link can operate only on a background of the senses, is capable of yielding only knowledge 'about' something, and must be differentiated from the O link essential to transformations in O. Before interpretations of hallucination can be given, which are themselves transformations O > K, it is necessary that the analyst undergoes in his own personality the transformation O > K. By eschewing memories, desires, and the operations of memory he can approach the domain of hallucinosis and of the 'acts of faith' by which alone he can become at one with his patients' hallucinations and so effect transformations O > K.

The pictorial representation of the dead man's shoes is a transformation of O in K, an experience which "phenomenalizes" into an image, an affective ideogram ([1992] 2014); an image which is in the hallucinosis scope for there is no sensory support in capturing this psychic reality. This happens through the analyst's intuition capacity, which evolves to a reverie, that is, it enters the field of representations.

We may ponder that, in the analyst's mind, upon the emotional turbulence of the encounter, a transformation from O to K occurred, that is to say, something formless (O) evolves to a form (K), a pictorial image. This is due to the analyst's reverie capacity, her α function – I remind you that the reverie is a factor of the α function, a function which transforms the brutality of the facts. K is a form, something that has "phenomenalized", it was susceptible to representation, through an image with aesthetics characteristics that can later be transformed by the analyst into a narrative, a verbal formulation, as Bion (1965) writes. In sum, O manifests itself in K (Bion [1970] 2014), "phenomenalizes" itself in K.

The aesthetical experience in the analytic session is another vertex emerging from *Transformations*. Bion describes the mutation done by the artist when painting a poppy field, and the invariants which makes the recognition of the poppy field possible. Still, this analogy will become more and more complex throughout the book. Would transformation in O be an aesthetic experience? Or would a transformation in K be it? Or could the hyperbolic distortions of projective transformations, and the transformation in hallucinosis be comprehended as aesthetic experiences? As we are usually in the face of pictorial constructions of the mind, the affective ideograms, an aesthetic experience seems to always be present in the several transformation vertexes, which could even be thought as aesthetic vertexes of the emotional experience.

The poetic language that Bion begins to use more frequently after *Transformations* and, undoubtedly, when he published *A Memoir of the Future* and his autobiographical texts, is a language of the aesthetic imagination, a language of achievement, as he wrote in *Attention and Interpretation* (1970). Only poetic language can be an evolution of transformations *in* O and *of* O. The mind organizes itself in *poiesis*, the waking dream capacity of dreaming the emotional experiences, an aesthetic, imaginative, constant and infinite creation.

Acknowledgements and history of *Reading Bion's Transformations*

'True novelty is that which does not grow old with the passing of time', becoming, perhaps, even better understood. This is the case, I believe, in Luís Cláudio Figueiredo's reading of *Transformations* in March 2000, having his graduate students at PUCSP as his interlocutors.

The moment at which those lessons took place is quite important, since very few papers referred to this shift in Bion's work during the 2000s. Particularly in regard to the statute of O, of Being and of become oneself, which is precisely examined in *Reading Bion's Transformations*, and what has been currently discussed amongst experts in Bion's work: the clinical statute of transformations in K and O.

In 2008, Gina Tamburrino and I were attending a PhD program and Luís Cláudio was our advisor. On that occasion he made his notes on the 2000 classes available to us so that we could organize a seminar on *Transformations*. We were greatly impacted by the originality and complexity of those notes and, without any hesitation, we remarked that it would be interesting to publish that material. Luís Cláudio invited us to organize and edit those precious notations and the book was published in Portuguese in 2011.

As a reference for the English-speaking reader, we find the book *Reading Bion*, by Rudi Vermote (2019) a good introduction to *Reading Bion's*

Transformations, which consists of a careful and detailed reading of one of Bion's theoretical books, considered extremely complex yet fundamental to consistently understand Bion's thinking.

The similarity in the book titles was not intentional – in Portuguese, title is *Bion in Nine Lessons: Reading Transformations*, and was published in 2011. The origin of this text lies in the seminars given by Luís Cláudio Figueiredo to his graduate students, hence we have kept the chapters numbered as lessons. The original title has a paradoxical, humorous character, since the book is not about introducing Bion in nine lessons, but about offering a complex reading of *Transformations* (1965). As a result, we decided to eliminate the first part of the original title here, which accentuates the proximity between the titles.

Apart from these coincidences, and as Bion puts is better himself: psychoanalytic thoughts seek authors in different geographic and psychic continents; the books are written in diverse languages and times; nevertheless, they can interconnect, even if only partially, in their textuality. Furthermore, the title in English allows a second comprehension: that Figueiredo follows closely the vestiges left by Bion of his own transformations as a thinker of psychoanalytic theory and as clinical practitioner, as mentioned before.

Finally, we would like to thank Luís Cláudio Figueiredo, who was generous in agreeing to publish his ideas for English-speaking readers; to my colleague Gina Tamburrino, who also supported the idea. To Elias da Rocha Barros for the preface to this English edition, and also for his enthusiasm for translating and publishing the book, which was fundamental. To Howard Levine for his interest in the ideas contained here and for his diligent orientation towards the writing of an introduction to guide the English-speaking reader in the challenges of reading the text – both the original text by Bion, *Transformations*, as well as the reading presented in this book.

Translating is, in part, a betrayal of the original text. Portuguese and English are languages with completely different structures, which makes the venture of translation both risky arduous. We thank Davi B. Flores, the translator, and Taís de O. Nicoletti, the translation editor, who accepted the challenge of translating to English an already difficult and complex book in its original language, Portuguese. They are psychoanalysts and researchers interested in Bion's work, and both take part in my research group at Universidade de São Paulo (USP) and at LipSic[11] (Interinstitutional Laboratory for Studies on Intersubjectivity and Contemporary Psychoanalysis IPUSP – PUCSP).

I thank Júlio Frochtengarten (2012) for the book review, written in Portuguese for the original edition, which was a reference for this text. I am grateful to the careful, attentive reading of this introduction's manuscript and for the suggestions made by Evelise Marra, Ignácio Gerber, Júlio Frochtengarten, and Gina Tamburrino.

I thank Evelise de Souza Marra, co-organizer of the conferences on Bion's work that have taken place in São Paulo since 2008, and which have been carried out with the collaboration of other colleagues from Sociedade Brasileira de Psicanálise de São Paulo (SBPSP) – Brazilian Psychoanalytic Society of São Paulo. To date there have been sixteen conferences and along with literature generated from these fruitful events (several papers and books), they maintain Bion's legacy in Brazil in constant expansion. And now, part of this consistent Brazilian production is presented to the English-speaking reader, with Howard Levine as editor.

Notes

1 Luís Cláudio Figueiredo begins many of his articles and lectures with this expression: "To begin with". By doing this we pay tribute to this proficient and prolific psychoanalyst and researcher. Translator's note: In Portuguese, the literal meaning of this expression is "to begin this conversation". We have adopted the expression "to begin with" in English to give the same sense of informality and friendliness between the author and readers.

2 I thank Júlio Frochtengarten (2012) for the book review, written in Portuguese for the original edition, which was a reference for my introduction to the English edition. I am grateful to the careful, attentive reading of this Introduction and for the suggestions made by Evelise de Souza Marra, Ignácio Gerber, Júlio Frochtengarten and Gina Tamburrino.

3 In *Reading Bion*, Vermote (2019), refers to this change as a caesura in the Bionian work, dividing his book into before and after the caesura, connecting life and work. Nevertheless, this is not a division done only by Vermote, we also found this idea in Bléandonu (1993) and Grotstein (2007), amongst others.

4 Luís Cláudio Figueiredo has published widely Portuguese, resulting in twenty-four books up to this moment; he is considered one of the most read, cited and referred to psychoanalysts by his peers. English-speaking readers will find articles by this author in scientific journals.

5 The full story of how this book came to be is told at the end of this introduction.

6 The terms transformation and invariance have their origins in mathematics.

7 I will return to the concept of transformation in hallucinosis in the clinical vignette discussion at the end of this introduction.

8 Vermote (2019, p. 166) considers that in *Attention and Interpretation* (1970 [2014]), Bion "… succeeded in integrating T (K) and T (O) as a dual track of psychic functioning and change".

9 T. N.: Neologism created by the authors.

10 If we strictly remain within a Bionian conceptualization, resistance refers to the unknown, that is, to the spectrum known-unknown, and to learn and not to learn from emotional experience. Also note that when referring to the dyad conscious-unconscious, Bion proposes the finite-infinite dyad.

11 Luís Cláudio Figueiredo is currently one of LipSic's academic advisors.

References

Bion, W.R. ([1965] 2014). Transformations. In: *The Complete Works of W.R. Bion, Vol. V*, ed. C. Mawson. London: Karnac Books, pp. 115–280.

Bion, Wilfred R. ([1965] 2014). Memory and Desire. In: *The Complete Works of W.R. Bion, Vol. VI*, ed. C. Mawson. London: Karnac Books.

Bion, Wilfred R. ([1967] 2014). Notes on Memory and Desire. In: *The Complete Works of W.R. Bion, Vol. VI*, ed. C. Mawson. London: Karnac Books.

Bion, Wilfred R. ([1970] 2014). Attention and Interpretation: A Scientific Approach to Insight in Psycho-Analysis and Groups. In: *The Complete Works of W.R. Bion, Vol. VI*, ed. C. Mawson. London: Karnac Books.

Bion, W.R. ([1992] 2014). Cogitations. In: *The Complete Works of W.R. Bion, Vol. XI*, ed. C. Mawson. London: Karnac Books, pp. 1–350.

Bléandonu, G. (1993). *Wilfred R. Bion. A vida e a obra 1897–1979 [Wilfred R. Bion: Life and Work, 1897–1979]*, trans. L.L. Hoory and M. Mortara. Rio de Janeiro: Imago Editora.

Cintra, E.U. and Ribeiro, M.F.R. (2018). *Por que Klein? [Why Klein?]* São Paulo: Escuta.

Figueiredo, L.C. (1999). *Palavras cruzadas entre Freud e Ferenczi [Crosswords between Freud and Ferenczi]*. São Paulo: Escuta.

Figueiredo, L.C. (2000). *Notes from Lectures*. São Paulo: PU-CSP.

Figueiredo, L.C., Tamburrino, G. and Ribeiro, M. (2011). *Bion em nove lições. Lendo Transformações [Bion in Nine Lessons: Reading* Transformations]. São Paulo: Editora Escuta.

Frochtengarten, J. (2012). Book Review: Bion em nove lições: lendo Transformações. *Revista Brasileira de Psicanálise*, 46(3): 229–232. Available at: http://pepsic.bvsalud.org/scielo.php?script=sci_arttext&pid=S0486-641X2012000300016 [accessed 25 May 2024].

Gerber, I. and Figueiredo, L.C. (2018). *Por que Bion? [Why Bion?]*. São Paulo: Zagodoni Editora.

Grotstein, J. (2007). *A Beam of Intense Darkness: Wilfred Bion's Legacy to Psychoanalysis*. London: Karnac Books.

Grotstein, J. (2019). Listening to and reading Bion. In: R. Vermote, *Reading Bion*, pp. 238–243. New York and London: Routledge.

Mawson, C. (2014). Introduction. In: *The Complete Works of W.R. Bion, Vol. VI*, ed. C. Mawson. London: Karnac Books.

Vermote, R. (2019). *Reading Bion*. New York and London: Routledge.

Zimerman, D. (2004). *Bion da Teoria à Prática. Uma leitura didática [Bion from Theory to Practice: A Didactic Reading]*. Porto Alegre: Artmed.

Initial considerations

Bion, his work and the book, *Transformations*

The work of Wilfred Ruprecht Bion (1897–1979) – like that of other great thinkers and practitioners of psychoanalysis – is a long and continuous exercise of singularization. All those who embarked on such journeys with the exception of Freud – though quite possibly, even in his case, things were not that different – naturally had to deal with the tension between loyalty and betrayal, between continuity and rupture, between repetition and creation. In Bion's case, however, the effort to raise psychoanalytic thinking and practice to new heights, and not just to new stages, is extremely intense and explicit.

The work of Wilfred Ruprecht Bion (1897–1979) – like that of other great thinkers and practitioners of psychoanalysis – is a long and continuous exercise of singularization. All those who embarked on such journeys with the exception of Freud – though quite possibly, even in his case, things were not that different – naturally had to deal with the tension between loyalty and betrayal, between continuity and rupture, between repetition and creation. In Bion's case, however, the effort to raise psychoanalytic thinking and practice to new *heights*, and not just to new stages, is extremely intense and explicit.

Bion intends to make an upward movement: it is not just about going further, deeper, or inwards, or moving towards greater complexity, as we find in Ferenczi, Melanie Klein and Fairbairn; it is about going higher, although without losing touch with the finer details of the terrain – the clinical phenomena. Otherwise, there would be the great risk of megalomania and arrogance,[1] of claiming to have reached the heights of divine wisdom; never getting completely rid of such risk. From this emerges a surprising rhetoric: Bion moves almost without mediation from the most abstruse mathematical abstractions to concrete statements; heard from patients in a given session, and then transcribed without any background story. The abstractions are often difficult to interpret and the "clinical examples", far from clarifying the theory and making it more intelligible, also often demand an enormous effort of interpretation due to the fragmentary nature of the elements offered.

The truth is that Bion did not always write like that. Initially, he followed the pattern of much more complete, concatenated, and trustworthy case reports; narratives that made much sense, based on annotations. They are

DOI: 10.4324/9781003476573-2

excellent texts and, to this day, they are very interesting for psychoanalytic clinic. However, when he published the most important works of his "first phase" (Bion [1967] 2014) in a compilation, he prefaced them with an "Introduction" and supplemented them with a lengthy "Commentary" in which his worldview into the status of the clinical material on psychoanalytic writing becomes quite clear. The clinical report never reproduces what is fundamental in a session. The essence of a session, like the essence of any emotional experience is, in fact, unreproducible and completely unrepresentable. We deal only with *phenomena*, not with the *thing itself*; we deal with results of multiple, chained and infinite *transformation* processes, never with the *origin* of these transformations. With regard to the clinical material presented in texts, at best it is a good fiction that communicates something that good theory could also do. These are only distinct modalities of transformation and it should not be assumed that "cases" are closer to reality than theories. In fact, in both modalities of transformation – theoretical and fictional – the essence of psychoanalysis has been set aside, or rather, merely suggested as what the reader should refer to beyond what is said and written.

In the mature works of the 1960s, when Bion accumulates his great theoretical framework – *Learning from Experience* ([1962] 2014), *Elements of Psycho-Analysis* ([1963] 2014) and *Transformations* ([1965] 2014) – he does not create fictions, neither does he tell us beautiful stories based on accurate annotations, narratives with a beginning, middle and end. His theoretical abstractions, the mathematical formulas, and the famous "grid",[2] as well as the elements extracted from the sessions – also considered abstractions – are present in the texts to awaken, mobilize, surprise, and not to be readily understood. All these elements are present to stimulate thought processes in the reader, not to provide answers or reassurance. As an epigraph for *Elements of Psycho-Analysis*, Bion adds a sentence by Maurice Blanchot: "La réponse est le malheur de la question." The answer is the misfortune of the question, and psychoanalysis is the exercise of questioning, not answering. Bion then remarks: "Or, as I understand it, the answer is the disease that kills curiosity." How to teach without killing curiosity?

What is, or what can be taught, about the so-called "transmission" of psychoanalysis? The word *ensinar* (T.N.: which means teaching, in English) comes from the Latin term *in-signare*. The root word "in" has two possibilities of comprehension and use. The first possibility is of negation, as in in-significant, and the second possibility is of "within", "in" or "inwards", as in in-signe, in-troduction or en-acting, with "in" turned into "en", as in "*ensinar*". In order for us to understand Bion's teaching of psychoanalysis, it is important to recover the etymological meaning of *in-signare: to take into the sign*. But, on the other hand, this also requires – and that goes against the recognized etymology of the word, yet it addresses a psychoanalytic issue much valued by him – the practice of thinking of the negative, whereby *in-signare* must be read as destitution of the sign, de-signify.

What can a sign be devoid of, if not its meaning? We will see below that the *negative capability*, which Bion takes from Keats, is one's ability to withstand uncertainty, mystery, and doubt. This ability to devoid the signs of their meanings, leaving them unsaturated and apt for infinite realizations, is characteristic of thought itself. Thinking occurs in the object's absence. The thought rises from the impossibility of contact with the object in its full presence; those who do not tolerate the object, do not think and do not develop the apparatus for thinking.

Teaching, in the sense of taking into the sign and also devoiding the signs from their meanings, summarizes this lesson of Bion and justifies its odd rhetoric. From a theoretical and stylistic point of view, this could be considered the main weapon against megalomania, against claims to know the truth and identification with God. Paradoxically, this complex and esoteric-biased rhetorical style, in which the most concrete elements – the patient or analyst's loose speech – become abstractions, and the most sophisticated abstractions (formulas) might become trivial things and tools, is permanently sliding toward a kind of madness made of arrogance, curiosity and stupidity. Perhaps that leads to a certain tendency towards obscurantism and even the incidence of some catastrophic episodes among Bion's followers.

But let us return to the position of Bion's work within the field of psychoanalysis. Bion does not call into question the link between the Freudian trunk and the Kleinian branch. However, developments and returns to "sources" are marked by such differences in style, emphases, angles, perspectives, etc., that one understands the pretension of many readers and followers of Bion – perhaps affected by lack of oxygen from the heights and from esotericism – that he has given psychoanalysis a new beginning, opening an incommensurable horizon to Freud and Melanie Klein, as pointed out by Symington and Symington (1999). This hyperbolic interpretation of distances between Bion on one hand, and Freud and Klein on the other, would not, however, be preferred by the author himself, and not out of modesty.

Bion was not at all modest about his ambitions and accomplishments, nor did he speak or write to anyone who could not keep up with him on his varied and sometimes wild journeys through the fields of philosophy, mathematics, arts and psychoanalysis. He always tended towards a certain megalomania and arrogance, as already mentioned. Moreover, hyperbolically accentuating the "theoretical disjunction between Bion and Freud/Klein" (Symington and Symington, 1999) has the advantage of preparing us for the unusual Bionian text, though it deprives us of the much more fruitful challenge of following him in his transferences, or rather, in his transformations of Freud and Melanie Klein. For Bion, the various psychoanalytic theories need to be understood as transformations of an unrepresentable clinical experience in itself. Likewise, the various readings of an author – such as Freud or Klein – are the result of different transformation processes since Freud and Klein themselves will never be reached. As we will see further ahead, transferences correspond to one of the transformation forms of great interest to psychoanalysis, although they are not the only ones, and perhaps not the most important ones.

The subject of the 1965 book is *transformations*. It was initially conceived, as seen in the introduction, as an achievement so well constructed that it would dispense of all support given in previous works, in which, much more clearly, Bion relies on Freud and Melanie Klein. Writing a self-sufficient book that owed nothing to another and totally escaped the intertextuality field already reveals the author's unreasonable ambition. But he resigns himself and, candidly, apologizes for the fact that he is publishing a book that does not succeed in making the others dispensable. He refers explicitly, however, only to the two other recently published books and says: "The other two books are therefore *still* necessary for the understanding of this one. I regret this ..." (Bion, [1965] 2014, p. 125, emphasis added). This is a "flaw" that readers can pass over if they are really interested in the thoughts expressed there, even if in an awkward way. The need to resort to other books is understood as accidental – a passing imperfection – and not as an expression of intertextuality. This aspect makes every book acquire meaning in its remission and in its parasitism of other books, of the author himself or others.

What underlies the supposed possibility of a book that dismisses others? Surely the belief in a transformation that brings us into contact with "reality", with "origin", objects as "things in themselves", what he will call the O of experience. One does not suppose – as it would be contradictory to the Bionian doctrine – that the book contains the knowledge of O. There cannot be adequate representation of O. However, there may be a "become O", and what the book may aspire to is the propitiation of passing from K (symbol that brings us to Knowledge) to O (symbol that brings us to Origin, One and Object). It would be the transition from *knowing about* to *becoming*.

Before moving on, it is important to remember that in some texts about Bion, O is translated as Zero. It seems that alongside L for Love, H for Hate, and K for Knowledge, it makes much more sense to postulate O as Origin, One, and Object. The *transition to O*, for example, is said to be *at-one-ment* and refers to *being at one with*. On the other hand, the word *at-one-ment* means expiation (atonement) and purification in the field of theology; reparation in the legal field, and reconciliation and concord in the social life field. The *at-one-ment*'s form of writing condenses the idea of *being one with oneself*, as opposed to *knowing oneself*, still marked by the dissociation in which "one knows and the other is", and the ideas of expiation, reparation and reconciliation. Such ideas underscore the experiences of being one with God and being with each other and with society after getting rid of sins and paying for crimes. *Becoming what one is* as an effect of analysis, involves all these operations. However, and we will return to this, Zero can signal an absence that helps us understand O as *the void and formless infinite* of the unconscious. In short, while there are strong reasons for keeping O as O, and not translating it as Zero, one must keep open the question of what O should mean. One of the possible interpretations could certainly lead to the notion of Zero. Only a close and deconstructive reading of the text may be capable of placing these different ways of referring to O, and yet probably will not lead to one single interpretation. At this point we can already anticipate one of the focuses of reading to be undertaken here: what are the statuses of O in the plane of transformations?

But we shall return to the theme of hope in the book that suffices itself. The book of books, the book that dismisses other books. *Transformations* would not be that book yet, but O is present in its horizons. The book would be able to induce this transition from K to O in the reader who, then, could count on his immediate experience of O, and would no longer need the experience of others transformed into speeches, texts, narratives and formulas, products of more or less successful transformations which, nevertheless, tend to accumulate like rubble in countless books.

It is not difficult to realize the extremes of obscurantism, hermeticism and megalomania that could result of a belief in the book that dismisses other books. One of the effects of this belief would be establishing a caste of *first readers of the book*, which might then spare its listeners and followers – even from this atoning sacrifice – by simply recommending: live, feel, intuit, think! Why study in false and ineffective books? But *Transformations*, according to Bion, is not yet this book, fortunately. And only for this reason we can read and take advantage of it.

Notes

1 Bion has made the themes – megalomania and arrogance – the focus of many works: "The meaning with which I wish to invest the term 'arrogance' may be indicated by supposing that in the personality where life instincts predominate, pride becomes self-respect, where death instincts predominate, pride becomes arrogance" (Bion, *Second Thoughts: Selected Papers on Psychoanalysis* [1967] 2014, p. 131).
2 The grid should be used to categorize uses and qualities of speeches in a session, from the point of view of the ongoing analytical process.

References

Bion, W.R. ([1962] 2014). Learning from Experience. In: *The Complete Works of W.R. Bion, Vol. IV*, ed. C. Mawson. London: Karnac Books, pp. 247–365.

Bion, W.R. ([1963] 2014). Elements of Psycho-Analysis. In: *The Complete Works of W.R. Bion, Vol. V*, ed. C. Mawson. London: Karnac Books, pp. 1–86.

Bion, W.R. ([1965] 2014). Transformations. In: *The Complete Works of W.R. Bion, Vol. V*, ed. C. Mawson. London: Karnac Books, pp. 115–280.

Bion, W.R. ([1967] 2014). Second Thoughts: Selected Papers on Psychoanalysis. In: *The Complete Works of W.R. Bion, Vol. VI*, ed. C. Mawson. London: Karnac Books.

Symington, J. and Symington, N. (1999). *O pensamento clínico de Wilfred Bion* [*The Clinical Thought of Wilfred Bion*]. Lisbon: Climepsi.

First lesson

Reading Chapter 1 of *Transformations*

The first chapter of *Transformations* takes up 11 pages, in which Bion introduces us immediately to the vast field of relations between "experiences" and their representations. We use quotation marks in "experiences", because the status of what is called "theme", "realization", "material", "facts" or "primitive experience" is far from being clear and univocally conceived.

The first chapter of *Transformations* takes up eleven pages, in which Bion introduces us immediately to the vast field of relations between "experiences" and their representations. We use quotation marks in "experiences", because the status of what is called "theme", "realization", "material", "facts" or "primitive experience" is far from being clear and univocally conceived:

> Suppose a painter sees a path through a field sown with poppies and paints it: at one end of the chain of events is the field of poppies, at the other a canvas with pigment disposed on its surface. We can recognize that the latter represents the former, so I shall suppose that despite the differences between a field of poppies and a piece of canvas, despite the transformation that the artist has effected in what he saw to make it take the form of a picture, *something* has remained unaltered and on this *something* recognition depends.
>
> (Bion [1965] 2014, p. 127)

What is the status of this "something"? In order to confront this issue, it is necessary to make some considerations. What the painter sees – the phenomenal origin of the painting – is certainly not unknowable, although it may be unknown to someone capable of interpreting the painting correctly, even observing it in the absence of the portrayed landscape. Seeing a trail across a field sown with poppies, or any other landscape endowed with form and meaning, already places us in the field of representations, that is to say, of the products of some transformation(s).

The painter can be sure that it is a landscape indeed, as he saw it, using other senses than sight; he can also share the "reality" of the landscape with a multitude of people. It is what Bion called *common sense*: the intra and intersubjective

DOI: 10.4324/9781003476573-3

correlation of meanings that guarantees a "reality" of what can be shared, published. In other words, a correspondence between the painting and the landscape implies the possibility of detecting homologies between the arrangement of the pigments on the canvas and the arrangement of the elements contained in the common sense view – or consensual view – of the landscape. The assumption that there is something that remains unchanged through invariants derives from consensual view. *Something* that can only be assumed from the recognition of a certain structural identity between the two poles in the chain.

Therefore, the two ends of the chain are on the same plane: the products of individual transformations – the painting by the painter – and collective – a common sense view of the landscape. Only the "something" would take us to another plane. This is important because, in this case, the transformation that serves as "origin" – the landscape recognized by all – is in fact more at the "social" end and less at the personal and singular end of this chain, the intersubjective pole. In several moments, it is possible to find, in this first chapter, the analogy that Bion makes between the transformation the painter makes by painting, and the transformation that the psychoanalyst makes when describing, narrating or theorizing an analytical session. In the second case, however, the movement does not seem to be the same, since the "experience" to be communicated requires the same evidence: it is not a previously structured object according to *common sense* criteria.

Let's go a little further. In the following paragraphs Bion presents the reader with some aspects of the transformations made by the painter: there is a perspective, for example, an angle of view, which determines the representation and the possibility of recognition. Invariants and their recognition – field of structural relations between elements – depend on the angle and technique adopted by the painter – on the "school" of painting to which he belongs – as well as on the previous conditions of those who will appreciate his work, that is, on the aesthetic and cultural experiences of those who see and interpret the painting. Likewise, psychoanalytical interpretations, narratives and theories would be transformations of the "experience of analyzing patients" from a certain angle and assuming the reader's singularity. Let us follow this paragraph:

> For my purpose it is convenient to regard psychoanalysis as belonging to the group of transformations. *The original experience*, the *realization* – in the instance of the painter the subject that he paints, and in the instance of the psychoanalyst the *experience of analysing* his patient – is *transformed* by painting in the one and analysis in the other into a painting and a psychoanalytic description respectively. The psychoanalytic interpretation given in the course of an analysis can be seen to belong to this same group of transformations. An interpretation is a transformation; to display the invariants, an experience felt and described in one way is described in another.[1]
>
> (Bion [1965] 2014, p. 129, emphasis added)

The question is whether there is equivalence between the painter's "subject" or "theme" – defined and built on the plane of common sense, which may be recognized by everyone as "a trail in a poppy field" – and the *original experience*. The *original experience*, be it that of the psychoanalyst who listens and feels his patient, or that of the painter himself who looks at the landscape, and from this plane both transform this "something" creating a painting or a verbal description which could be recognized as corresponding to that "something". In the case of the analyst, it seems that it would effectively mean a "creation", and not just a transformation from one representation into another. In fact, the term *realization*, adopted by Bion for both "theme" and "experience of analyzing", is ambiguous, as it can be literally considered *something made real*. Bion suggests that any *realization* is no longer the original experience, as this is unknowable, but rather the creative product of a given transformation (of the original experience). However, in the text they appear as synonyms.

At the end of the following paragraph, Bion reaffirms the analogy between the painter who by painting transforms the landscape and the psychoanalyst who theorizes and interprets:

> For my present purpose it is helpful to regard psychoanalytic theories as belonging to the category of groups of transformations, a technique analogous to that of a painter, by which the facts of an analytic experience (the realization) are transformed into an interpretation (the representation). Any interpretation belongs to the class of statements embodying invariants under one particular psychoanalytic theory ...
>
> (Bion [1965] 2014, p. 130)

The analogy with the painter is taken up and another dimension is added to it: the equivalence between the technique or school of a painter – for example, the impressionist – and the theory or school of a psychoanalyst – for instance, the Kleinian. In a footnote Bion will say, for example, that *in clinical practice* we do not want to talk about "Kleinian transformations" as opposed to "Freudian transformations". This observation implies that the analyst in his work produces transformations much less committed to any technique or theory, but more dependent on his perception, with regard to the demands of the clinical situation. From a conceptual point of view, however, this mode of expression would make sense.

The passage transcribed above also adds something to the supposed equivalence between experience and realization: the notion of "facts". If an experience is made up of facts – and he does not use quotes to refer to facts – it can surely be equivalent to a realization. So that there are "facts" and "recognition of facts", some work of symbolization has already occurred creating identifiable elements, that means, endowed with some form and some sense, and might be wholly experienced. But, in this case, the condition of transformation product that is attributed to the experience itself becomes even clearer. As for the Bionian notion of "indigestible facts", it is used to refer to the raw ingredients of the experience prior to any processing and before its inclusion in the psyche. Such a notion should not be understood in banal terms; these facts are unlike any other. The true nature of "indigestible facts" is as obscure and disconcerting as that of "something" that remains unchanged throughout the transformations.

Continuing with Bion's text, we highlight that psychoanalytic theories are presented as transformations of experience – realizations – capable of generating other transformations, the interpretations. The origin – the painting's theme, facts of clinical experience – both implies transformation and generates transformations (theories) capable of giving rise to determined classes of transformations: interpretations, whether Kleinian, Freudian, Winnicottian, etc. To that extent, the distinction between realization and representation loses all clarity, both implying a process of transformation.

On the other hand, there are representations produced at very different levels and processes, for example, theories and interpretations. Not only do they originate from previous transformations, they are also the origin of new transformations. This seems obvious in the case of theories – true machines of transformation – but also of interpretations that, in order to be clinically effective, must necessarily be capable of generating transformative effects.

Following the text, we will see that Bion introduces another term to refer to the origins of the transformations:

> Kleinian transformation, associated with certain Kleinian theories, would have different invariants from those in a classical Freudian transformation. Since the invariants would be different, so the meaning conveyed would be different even if the *material* transformed (the analytic experience or realization) could be conceived of as being the same in both instances.
> (Bion [1965] 2014, p. 131, emphasis added)

Imagining the "material" as being "the same", that is, as being subject to the principle of identity, presupposes that the "material" must necessarily be taken as the product of some transformation. More than that: it must exist at the level of common sense and be shareable. The term "material" has since reappeared several times in the chapter:

> The analyst's main concern must be with the material of which he has direct evidence; ... The analyst gives interpretations, when they appear to be appropriate to the *material*; ... The material lends itself to interpretations based on Kleinian theories; ... In this situation the analyst must search the *material* for invariants to the pre- and post-catastrophic stages; ... Restating this in terms of clinical *material* ...
> (Bion [1965] 2014, p. 133 and 134, emphasis added)

Insofar as the facts of the experience, realizations, theme and subject and, in particular, clinical material are used interchangeably, there is nothing to suggest that what is at the origin of a transformation is of a different nature from the product of a transformation. Everything leads us to believe that the supposed *something*, from the invariants, is not at the origin, but in the middle of the transformations. In fact, the term "material" is associated with the notion of evidence, with the idea of correspondence or adequacy (*interpretations appropriate to the material*), with the assumption of structure (*invariants must be sought in the material*). Everything, therefore, suggests the existence of a form already present in the "material". Hence, none of this could lead us to expect Bion's postulation, not expressed until this part of the text, that the experiential origin of the transformations is unknowable in itself. For now, we are moving between transformations and never going beyond them and their products. The *something* that remains in the invariants of different transformations, far from being the basis of transformations, would be what can be deduced from the fact that they apparently correspond.

After this arid traverse through philosophical questions, the reader could ask himself: what does this have to do with psychoanalysis? Bion replies:

> Throughout this book I suggest a method of critical approach to psychoanalytic practice and not new psychoanalytic theories. By analogy with the artist and the mathematician I propose that the work of the psychoanalyst should be regarded as transformation of a realization (the actual psychoanalytic experience) into an interpretation or series of interpretations.
>
> (Bion [1965] 2014, p. 131)

The distinction between a critical approach of practice and a theory is that the first is placed simultaneously and paradoxically closer and farther from experience. Closer, because it intends to show the main features of the structure and dynamics involved in the experience of psychoanalytic practice. Farther, because it necessarily places itself at a level of universality and abstraction higher than that of theories. A critical approach to psychoanalytic practice presupposes that it can be identified at a higher level than the theories that differ from one another and conflict with each other. There is, therefore, in the renunciation of a new theory – which is not quite true, because in previous books and texts, Freud and Klein are submitted to innumerable creative transformations – more pretension than modesty. The intention is to position itself on the plane of what would be a metatheory which, however, does not deal with theories, but, going through them, returns directly to the field of clinical experience. Since then, it is possible to understand the twofold dimension of the Bionian text: split between the most intricate abstractions, of strong philosophical and mathematical nature, and the details of a session or a clinical case. And, also, the ambition to write a book that dispenses with other books, and that makes critical contact with clinical experience without the mediation of psychoanalytic theories. Following the Bionian text:

> Psychotic mechanisms appear in the course of a psychoanalytically controlled breakdown, but the analyst may be called upon to deal with them after such a breakdown has occurred, or, because something has happened, despite the work of the analyst, to precipitate such a breakdown during analysis.
>
> (Bion [1965] 2014, p. 132)

The following paragraph makes Bion's speech particularizing: "The man could be regarded, in view of the predominance of psychotic mechanisms and bizarre behaviour, as a borderline psychotic" (Bion [1965] 2014, p. 132). The next one is even more surprising. Without further introduction he begins: "Then a change: friends or relations who have been denying that there is anything the matter cannot ignore his illness" (Bion [1965] 2014, p. 132). There is very brief information below about what was happening with the patient. In fact, the case in its singularity does not matter much and, moreover, is left open. However, the effect of a sudden introduction to such a heterogeneous argument in comparison to what was being woven in a high plane of abstractions, reproduces in the plane of writing the collapse that the text causes. There is something catastrophic about this rhetoric, and it is precisely about catastrophe what Bion will deal with.

First, an event is catastrophic if it generates a system or order subversion. Second, if it is accompanied by feelings of disaster. Third, if it is sudden and violent in an almost physical way. Bion's interest is in showing that in pre- and post-catastrophic states invariants can be identified. These attest that it is the same analysis, although numerous changes have occurred: in tone, colour, and affective intensity. In the post-catastrophic stages certain mechanisms, hitherto operating silently, become noisy and evident. However, it is the same mechanisms that remain under change, as specific operators of that analysis.

At this point in the Bionian text, the issue of transformations reaches a higher level of complexity. We have to consider both the transformations of relatives and friends that detect something in the "material" offered by the patient, developing lay ideas, and the analyst's transformations that are based on his experiences with the analysand and, mainly, the transformations before and after the collapse. These transformations can, for example, turn hypochondriac pains into delusions, although preserving something invariant. Persecutory phantasies arise where the knee pains were; they are a transformation of pain in the post-catastrophic period.

It is from this crossover of transformations that invariants can emerge – something that remains – but we still do not realise the status of what would be transformed first and foremost; of the object itself before a transformation, that is, we know nothing about the origin of the transformations. In order to deal with this shuffling of transformations and their remaining invariants, which could be expressed, Bion feels the need to qualify them. First, the term is divided into three: Transformations (T) encompass transformations in terms of process (T α) and transformations in terms of products (T β).

To be understood, these denominations compel us – which is a shame! – to consult other books. Beginning with Chapter 3 of *Learning from Experience* (1962), Bion proposes that the most primitive elements of experience, prior to any symbolization, should be named elements β. Such elements require symbolization, that is, a metabolic process capable of converting them into thoughts themselves: they are like elements of a protomental system (Symington and Symington, 1999, p. 84). Therefore, they cannot enter and, even less, remain in the psyche. In the absence of a device (one's own, or someone else's) to think about them, they – as indigestible facts – will be evacuated. This is what happens under the dominance of the pleasure principle – postulated by Freud – in which the only path to relief is that of immediate reduction of tension, the accumulation of indigestible facts, through evacuation release. The β elements are themselves unknowable and non-storable. It is the transformation process that digests and symbolizes them, converting them into α elements that can be stored and used by the psyche. The function of transforming β elements into α elements is called α function.[2]

It is clear, from these theorizations, that for Bion the problem of transformations was present even though it was not the main focus of his writings. The α function is, obviously, a transformation function. However, given the unknowable nature of the β elements, and the fact that Bion can only reach them by a transcendental deduction – *à la* Kant – the α function is, actually, creative and never reproductive. It responds, supposedly, to a demand imposed by the β elements, also supposed, constituting the α elements, coequally hypothetical, those who could effectively take shelter in the psyche. An observation should be made here: even when the α function does not work and the β elements are evacuated – through psychosomatic symptoms, hallucinations or delusions and acting-outs, for example, what is found is no longer the β elements in themselves, but products of some transformation.

Let us return to the book *Transformations*. It is not surprising that the transformation processes are called T α, although the α function used to refer to a transition from the condition of thing itself (β elements) to the condition of primitive thought. Now, all transitions, including evacuation transitions, are recognized as containing and implying some transformation – for example, transformation into hallucinosis. The sign α refers now to the whole transformation process.

On the other side, the products of these processes are called T β. Formerly, the β elements were deduced and supposed to be at the almost psychic/almost corporeal origin of psychic life. They were elements that, like Freud's *drives*, were at the limits between psychic and somatic. The ingredients of this pro-tomental system, in which the somatic and the psychic are still undiffer-entiated, would not be hosted in the mind, in a thinking apparatus, but spread throughout the body and the interfaces between the somatic and the psychic. They are the sense impressions, whether directly produced by the external environment, or mainly those derived from affections, emotions. Sense impressions are fundamentally what characterize the somatic dimension of affects, being the term closer to our notion of sensuality than to sensoriality, in which the affective dimension is attenuated. When the mind is not prepared to think these proto-thoughts (affections, or rather, affective intensities in a raw state), they will demand a foreign mind, as is the case of the relationship between baby and mother. In this situation, a mother's capacity for reverie performs the α function for the child. The mother thinks the proto-thoughts (affective intensities, "sensualities") disseminated in the baby's body and evacuated to her own body (by projective identification), to then return them gradually to the infant – more elaborated, well thought out – constituting into the child, progressively, an apparatus for self-thinking.

In *Transformations*, the reference to β elements reappears, but after a transformation process when they exist as T β. In fact, this is the "material" that someone provides to others – and to himself – to start a new sequence of transformations. As a product of a transformation, it already has some form and meaning, even if very primitive. But as a source of new transformations, this "material" is, like the β elements, unknowable in itself.

Therefore, there is a double condition: on one hand, the β elements are assumed from a transcendental deduction without ever showing themselves; on the other hand, transformations generate empirically verifiable products (they do not need to be assumed, nor deduced) and endowed in some way with meaning, but they trigger and demand new cycles of transformation and, in a sense, are unknowable in themselves.

In order for the intricate, intersecting chains of transformations to be understood, Bion feels the need to indicate their "vehicle". That is why it is necessary to attach to the abbreviations an indication of who is supporting the transformation. T (patient) α refers to the patient's transformation pro-cesses from where T (patient) β originates, which will be, in turn, the trigger-ing "material" for T (analyst) α which will consecutively be the generators, for example, of interpretations that will have the status of T (analyst) β.

This may all seem too strange to the reader, but it is important to underline some aspects. Although a transcendental origin of transformations may be supposed from the invariants, and from that "something" which remains, we are always actually dealing with chained transformations and their products, but never with the thing itself in its full presence.

On the other hand, and as a result, transformations are never inevitable effects of what triggered them; that is, between the supposed "origin" and the subsequent transformation there are not causal relationships prevailing: the same material (T (patient) β) will lead family members, friends, the analyst – and even some other analyst with a different orientation or with different experience and sensitivity – to completely distinct transformation processes. This is because T (patient) β, although already endowed with some form and meaning for being the product of certain transformation, has a β dimension, that is, it is partly unknowable, enigmatic, bizarre. The more disturbed and primitive a communication is, the more obscure it will be, and the more open will be the alternatives for transformation.

Altogether, the proposed idea is that we are permanently moving between processes and products of transformations, not being able to rely definitively on any empirical or even transcendental support, although a remission to transcendence may emerge through the deduction that *something* must exist at the origin of everything and of all transformations. However, this *something* has in no way the apparent simplicity of a painting's theme, as it is suggested to us at the beginning of the chapter. The "clinical material" – even though it already contains some forms and patterns from which invariants can be extracted (as Bion suggests) – is far from having the closure and univocity capable of determining, once and for all, the most appropriate psychoanalytic transformation, the proper interpretation. This "material"[3] contains a β, enigmatic, intrusive, disturbing dimension, which compels us to work, but does not fully determine what to do with it: the T (patient) β. It seems complicated, it seems very risky, nevertheless:

> If the reader considers the first chapter in the light of his experience he will realize that any apparent strangeness lies in the method of approach and not in the experience described. It will help understanding if he will satisfy himself before he reads further that phenomena described are already familiar to him.
>
> (Bion [1965] 2014, p. 136)

And this is how Bion ends the first chapter of the book *Transformations*.

Notes

1 In general, by the patient, but also by the analyst, if we consider their counter-transference impacts.
2 It is worth sharing a brief explanation: the use of letters and abbreviations is due to the attempt to escape saturation of meaning which concepts usually carry with their associative penumbra. By calling the elements α and β Bion seeks to express himself in a less ladened, less saturated and more abstract way, becoming, therefore, more apt to mathematical and free thinking.
3 Although the name is so reassuring, "matter" is made of the same Latin root that gives us "mother", *mater*.

References

Bion, W.R. ([1965] 2014). Transformations. In: *The Complete Works of W.R. Bion, Vol. V*, ed. C. Mawson. London: Karnac Books, pp. 115–280.

Symington, J. and Symington, N. (1999). *O pensamento clínico de Wilfred Bion* [*The Clinical Thought of Wilfred Bion*]. Lisbon: Climepsi.

Second lesson

Reading Chapter 2 of *Transformations*

The following two chapters (2 and 3) of Bion's *Transformations* have a very close relationship with each other. The second chapter is structured in three easily identifiable parts. First, Bion takes up the problem of transformations abstractly. Second, he presents the clinical material that will support the analysis and definition of what he calls rigid motion transformation, corresponding to transference. Finally, he presents clinical material of another nature, which should not be understood as transference but rather in terms of projective transformation. The clinical material is not analyzed at this time. The analysis of this process will take place in Chapter 3, so only then will the distinction between both modalities of transformation become more understandable, and, therefore, the clinical difference between neurosis and psychosis will begin to be established, as announced in the second chapter. Considering that there is an intimate connection between both chapters, it would be interesting to read them sequentially, afterward taking them up and analyzing each one in its theoretical and rhetorical details.

The following two chapters (2 and 3) have a very close relationship with each other. The second chapter is structured in three easily identifiable parts. At first Bion takes up the problem of transformations in an abstract way. Second, he presents the clinical material that will support the analysis and definition of what he calls *rigid motion transformation*, corresponding to transference. Finally, he presents clinical material of another nature, which should not be understood as transference, but rather in terms of projective transformation. The clinical material is not analyzed at this time. The analysis of this process will take place in Chapter 3, so only then will the distinction between both modalities of transformation become more understandable and, therefore, the clinical difference between neurosis and psychosis will begin to be established, as announced in the second chapter.

Considering that there is an intimate connection between both chapters, it would be interesting to read them sequentially, afterwards taking them up and analyzing each one in its theoretical and rhetorical details. Two sentences draw the attention: the first opens the second chapter and the second is at the end of the third:

DOI: 10.4324/9781003476573-4

The term 'transformation' may mislead unless the limitations of the implication of 'form' are recognized.

(Bion [1965] 2014, p. 137)

... we must be prepared to find the model of the painter misleading though still useful.

(Bion [1965] 2014, p. 157)

Both sentences show limitations and the potential to mislead contained in forms of expression and analogies which have been selected and constructed, which in addition are useful and, in some ways, inevitable. What word could advantageously replace the term *transformation*? These moments of explicit recognition of the precariousness of communications are corroborated by the frequent use of expressions, such as: *in other words, in other terms, putting it in another way*, without ever reaching the proper expression. This way of using a language – due to lack of alternatives – that always falls short of what is necessary and, therefore, must be infinitely unfolded in analogies, metaphors, stylistic novelties, formulas, etc, reminds us of Hillis-Miller's logic of "not only, but instead", also recognized in Freud and Ferenczi (Figueiredo, 1999). In Bion's case, this quality of language insufficiency is clearly based on his Kantian assumption that it is impossible to access the thing-in-itself, that is, the external fact or episode, or the experience itself, or the psychic transformations of external reality or, even, the results of these transformations etc. (Bion [1965] 2014, pp. 137 and 138). As we shall see, not only does the status of O – the origin of transformations – oscillate, but the unknowable thing-in-itself lurks at every step. We are surrounded by unknowns and unknowables. However, for precisely this reason, we continue to speak, since we have no other way!

The term *transformation* suggests that we are dealing with forms, such as moving from one form to another. The painter's model assumes that a common sense form – the landscape – becomes indeed a more personal one – the painting, although there are invariants that allow it to be recognized as the landscape's representation. In painting, and in geometry, it makes sense to think in these terms, as Bion confirms. Yet he warns: "I am concerned with a function of personality in the process of being represented and it may introduce errors to suppose that a function of personality *has* a form" (Bion [1965] 2014, p. 137, emphasis added). From *misleading* to *misleading* we come across the highly deceptive term *personality* and, even worse, *function of personality*. What would we have as an alternative? Freud had already adopted the term in the 31st lecture in *New Introductory Lectures on Psychoanalysis* ([1932] 1933), entitled "The Dissection of the Psychical Personality" [Die Zeregungung psychischen Persönlichkeit]. To mention one more example, we cite W.R.D. Fairbairn's *Psychoanalytic Studies of the Personality* (1952). In both cases the term was removed from its common use, in which personality is associated with the notion of unity – an individual unity – to be later decon-structed. In place of the unitary personality we have, in Freud, the decom-position of this unit in the second topic instances and, in Fairbairn, an even more complex topic in terms of splits and dissociations. In each case it is necessary to say something and then take it back, saying it again in a different way, yet likewise unsatisfactory.

Returning to the text, the expression *function of personality* is justified in the first chapter of *Learning from Experience* ([1962] 2014). Bion starts, as always, with what is most obvious and seemingly natural. There is no doubt when he says that this or that action, being typical in the conduct of a given individual, can be understood as a function of his personality. He says:

> I take advantage of this usage to derive a theory of functions that will stand up to more rigorous use than that for which the conversational phrase is employed. I shall suppose that there are factors in the personality that combine to produce stable entities which I call functions of the personality.
>
> (Bion [1962] 2014, p. 269)

Soon afterwards Bion clarifies the meanings of *factor* and *function* using examples. The observable field – behaviour and speech – is supposedly deter-mined by sets of inferred factors that constitute functions, these also being inferred. That way, one could only access the product of a mental activity (function) which, in turn, is composed of conjugated elements (factors). Then he presents the function that will be his main object of examination, the α function, written integrally as alpha-function in *Learning from Experience*, as well as α and β elements will be spelled *alpha* and *beta elements*. In the fol-lowing book, *Elements of Psycho-Analysis*, the Greek alphabet is adopted, giving the discourse an even stranger physiognomy. These are small details that must not go unnoticed. In *Learning from Experience* ([1962] 2014) Bion adopts symbols: L for *Love*, H for *Hate*, K for *Knowledge* and ♀ ♂ to refer to the container-contained relationship. However, the introduction of α and β adds more elements to a discourse's production tending towards abstract notations. As always, they are attempts of critical – and ironic – use of col-loquial language that can neither be overcome nor be easily used.

Resuming our proposal, that is, to understand what Bion means by *function of personality*, it is possible to find there, preformed, a theory of transforma-tions. *Personality* is not a unitary entity, neither stable nor substantial. It is instead a place where factors are brought together to exercise functions, whose products are "material" available to possible observations. In saying that personality functions have no form, Bion is trying to withdraw what he involuntarily, but inevitably, suggests. He needs to discard the belief that per-sonality is a form, and that its products, actions and works are transforma-tions – reproductions – of an original form. Nevertheless, these functions and combinations of factors are formative, creating more or less recognizable and decipherable forms. Severely ill patients often create forms that, at first sight, could be called deformations, as we cannot easily recognize their similarity to what may have been the original experience. Let us analyze, then, the last sentences of this first paragraph:

> Suppose that T_2 (patient) β is a shapeless lump, the term 'deformation' is not likely to mislead. But if T_2 (patient) α is the patient's experience of being greeted by the analyst, and T_2 (patient) β is the patient's representation of the event as a hostile attack made on him by the doctor, it may seriously obstruct understanding of what has taken place in the mind of the patient to suppose that either T_2 α or T_2 β have, or are, forms.
>
> (Bion [1965] 2014, p. 137)

The whole issue of invariants that was apparently well clarified in the relation between landscape and painting – which are effectively forms – is again obscure, which is a pity! It seemed so simple to understand the equivalence between forms, calling x, or *something* that remains; both to place x in the place of transcendence and to place it in the world of forms – a form among forms. If on the one hand understanding is lost, on the other hand certain theoretical freedom is gained: instead of *forms* we find *uses, processes, factors* and *functions*. A deconstruction of identity assumptions embedded in the notion of form is carried out, introducing a temporal dimension. One cannot have everything at once! Thinking advances renouncing what was already considered satisfactory as knowledge. Let us try to accompany him by detaching ourselves from everything that we so easily thought we had learned so far. Symington and Symington (1999) say that understanding Bion requires necessarily forgetting Freud and Melanie Klein. In part, that is an overstatement. Moreover, this is also insufficient: in order to understand Bion, it is necessary to forget Bion, to accompany him *without memory and desire*, along the paths he is exploring, step by step. We must be prepared to recognize that the simplest models and the easiest understandings are misleading, although useful.

At this moment, changing the direction of his journey, Bion resorts to the grid, the work presented in *Elements of Psycho-Analysis*:

> The Grid in *Elements of Psycho-Analysis* affords a method of escape from the implications of 'form' through resort to signs for abstract categories (the various grid compartments) to represent the content of T_2 α and T_2 β.
>
> (Bion [1965] 2014, p. 137)

Before exemplifying the use of his grid, Bion discusses issues that require attention:

> A sign to represent the realization would denote, to take the example in Chapter 1, the landscape as a thing- in-itself, and therefore distinguish it

from both $T_2\ \alpha$ and $T_2\ \beta$. The sign would denote something that is not a mental phenomenon and therefore, like Kant's thing-in-itself to make clear the status of $T_2\ \alpha$ and $T_2\ \beta$ as signs for mental phenomena.

(Bion [1965] 2014, p. 137)

At the beginning of the following paragraph, already introducing an example, Bion follows up the discussion on the thing-in-itself:

The use of these signs may be clarified by an illustration: The patient enters and, following a convention established in the analysis, shakes hands. This is an external fact, what I have called a 'realization'. In so far as it is useful to regard it as a thing-in-itself and unknowable (in Kant's sense) it is denoted by the sign O. The phenomenon, corresponding to the external fact, as it exists in the mind of the patient, is represented by the sign T (patient) α.

(Bion [1965] 2014, pp. 137–138)

Before proceeding with the reading of the paragraph in which Bion introduces the use of his grid, a few considerations are worth noting. In this moment the equivalence is: between a handshake understood as an external fact and as a *realization*, and the thing-in-itself as O. In contrast, there is the equivalence between the phenomenon – which corresponds to the external fact – as it exists in the patient's mind. Let us put aside the Bionian ambition to join Kant and the supposition that all this postulation is Kantian. However, we must question the consistency of the equations: how can a handshake – which implies action and reciprocity – be understood as an "external fact"? How can a conventional and perfectly recognizable and nameable act be taken as the unknowable thing-in-itself? Is it not, by contrast, a strong candidate for the status of phenomenon? How can T (patient) α – a transformation process – be taken as phenomenon if, strictly speaking, this process as such is what is never seen in itself, but only through its products T (patient) β? Even to the patient – or to anyone else – T α cannot show or exist as a phenomenon. Is he not a strong candidate for the status of unknowable? Precisely, would that not be the reason for demanding a sign devoid of meaning for its "representation", such as T α?

The purpose is neither to point out the inconsistencies and paralogisms in Bion's discourse, nor to question his supposed Kantianism, but to recognize two aspects of the passage quoted above. First, there is an emphasis, even though arbitrarily attributed, to the dimensions of unknowability that are present in all elements of experience, even in the most banal and everyday ones, like shaking hands. Second, it is worth noting that the heterogeneity of elements prevents that all sequences are placed on the same plane. Between the handshake and the mental processing of this episode, there is a small or large gap, but never a direct and immediate transition. In each of the "stages" – O, T α and T β – there is more, or less, of reality and meaning that prevents the formation of merely logical and obvious chains. In the same chapter, Bion will say that we are always searching for relations among three unknowns. Each of them contains its own unknowable and, to that extent, O infiltrates the entire chain. On the other hand, the *origin* – as in the case of the handshake, agreed and recognized – is never quite the thing-in-itself, the unknowable O, but it is necessarily a *realization*, something that can be seen, that phenomenalizes, but always harbouring in itself what cannot be shown.

The distinction between O, T α and T β helps to understand Bion but it also hinders it, since it unduly locates the unseen in the origin O. The unknowable does not appear only there – in the origin – in a pure state, nor is it excluded from all the other moments. We are surrounded by unknowns, and we live so mobilized in the effort to face them, as we inevitably generate new unknowns, including those generated by personal efforts to face the unknown. The signs adopted by Bion are justified by the need to maintain the clear notion that obscurity cannot be dispelled, nor should it be, and that the whole theoretical apparatus must not give the illusion that we already know something. On the contrary, the theoretical apparatus needs to be built to remind us of the unknown and send us back to it.

Having made these considerations, let us return to the Bionian text:

> This sign I mean to replace by a grid category. The grid category is determined by picking on that category to which my clinical observation of the patient's behaviour seems most closely to approximate. Suppose the handshake is intended as a denial of hostility that the patient experienced in a dream about me. His action would then fall in a category in column 2 and row C. The sign then would be C2.
>
> (Bion [1965] 2014, p. 138)

When faced with this type of presentation, the impact could not be greater or more disconcerting. First, Bion mentions the *patient's behaviours* as observable and classifiable in almost behaviorist terms. However, contrary to what a behaviorist would do, there is much speculation: it is possible to observe behaviours, but *the pretension to deny hostility* is not observable. It is an interpretation. So far, the impact is not so strong except for the Bionian discourse in which seemingly incompatible notions are mixed up, such as *observable behaviour and denial of hostility experienced in dreams*. In any case, interpreting certain phenomena as denial is no surprise to a psychoanalyst, who is used to working with phantasies, and not with behaviour in a strict sense. The following questions remain: how to reach this interpretation from a behaviour, and even more, from a conventional behaviour? What is the gain of – after the interpretation was made – registering it in grid's terms? Why transform *handshakes, like a fantasized denial of a dreamed hostility*, in C2?

The first question is answered next: "The associations following this start to the session would have yielded the evidence for choosing the sign C2" (Bion [1965] 2014, p. 138). Interpretations are, as always, based on associations, not behaviours, and are formed *a posteriori*. Categorization is subsequent to interpretive work based on associations. In fact, according to Bion, the grid should be used after a session, so that it does not spare the analyst from the work of analysis, also preventing a mechanical use of it. Even so, the other question remains: what is gained from categorizing, in terms of the grid, what resulted from the analyst's interpretations?

The start of an answer has been given: "The Grid in *Elements of Psycho-Analysis* affords a method of escape from the implications of 'form' through resort to signs for abstract categories" (Bion [1965] 2014, p. 137). This is, undoubtedly, a source of discontent for psychoanalysts when faced with the categorizations of the grid: very abstract, very disincarnated. Transforming a handshake, which in the phantasy is the denial of a dreamed hostility, in C2, causes an understandable reluctance to accept such a categorization. On the other hand, it is necessary to escape from the assumption of form when we acknowledge that even in the phenomena endowed with form and meaning there is something that cannot be seen, that does not phenomenalize and, therefore, is devoid of predetermined form and meaning. C2 says nothing, has no meaning of its own, and is in an unsaturated state, waiting for a meaning. This would be one reason for using the grid: the intuiting of the unknowable that inhabits the entire field of phenomena, and which forces us to give up the assumption of form. There are other advantages, and there are also risks which will become clear below. Beforehand, however, we must accompany Bion's text to the end of the paragraph:

> In addition I expect to find evidence on which to determine the category in which I shall place the representation that has resulted from his transformation, T, of the episode, O (thing-in-itself), to T (patient) α and thence to T (patient) β – this last being the representation, his representation, of the episode. This sign T (patient) β I shall now replace, as I have already done with T (patient) α, by a grid category. Once more the grid category must be determined by assessment of the associations. Suppose the evidence suggests that the patient's experience is that my handshake was a sexual assault on him. The context shows me that this approximates to a definitory hypothesis; I expect accordingly to find the category in column 1. If, from my knowledge of him, I am convinced that the patient is not experiencing this as a thought or idea or even as a dream, but as an actual fact, I assess the category to lie in row A – the β-elements. The category with which I replace T (patient) β is A1.

(Bion [1965] 2014, p. 138)

To know that T (patient) α can be C2 and T (patient) β can be A1 is not enlightening; it can even be less tranquilizing for a psychoanalyst. Containing and enduring this disquiet seems interesting, considering the observation made earlier about Bion's teaching as *in-signare*. To resume: the interpretation of the Latin word *in-signare* as *taking into the sign* and, simultaneously, *removing the signs from their meanings* in order to *en-sinar* ("teaching" in Portuguese), without killing curiosity. We believe that now the experience of this "teaching" can begin to be properly appreciated.

References

Bion, W.R. ([1962] 2014). Learning from Experience. In: *The Complete Works of W. R. Bion, Vol. IV*, ed. C. Mawson. London: Karnac Books, pp. 247–365.

Bion, W.R. ([1963] 2014). Elements of Psycho-Analysis. In: *The Complete Works of W. R. Bion, Vol. V*, ed. C. Mawson. London: Karnac Books, pp. 1–86.

Bion, W.R. ([1965] 2014). Transformations. In: *The Complete Works of W.R. Bion, Vol. V*, ed. C. Mawson. London: Karnac Books, pp. 115–280.

Fairbairn, W.R.D. (1952). *Psychoanalytic Studies of the Personality*. London: Routledge & Kegan Paul, 1981.

Freud, S. ([1932] 1933). Lecture XXI: The Dissection of the Psychical Personality. New Introductory Lectures on Psycho-Analysis. In: *The Standard Edition of the Complete Psychological Works of Sigmund Freud, Vol. XXII(1932–1936)*, trans. J. Strachey. London: The Hogarth Press and the Institute of Psychoanalysis.

Symington, J. and Symington, N. (1999). *O pensamento clínico de Wilfred Bion* [*The Clinical Thought of Wilfred Bion*]. Lisbon: Climepsi.

Third lesson

Continuing reading

The thing-in-itself was the external fact, the episode of shaking hands, which had already puzzled us. Now, the thing-in-itself is the "experience." The mental process of transforming the thing-in-itself into a phenomenon – T α – is now referred to as "impression." Now, the term "impression" refers us to an action of the object on the subject, keeping the subject in the passive (receptive) condition, while T α has suggested an activity so far, a processing engendered by the subject and exercised on the objects. Even in the following sentence, it is clearly stated that the representation results from the transformation the patient "made," emphasizing his activity and, therefore, making the identification of T α with the "impression" even stranger.

Let us return, then, to the question of transformations in the Bionian text:

> Using the facts (of my illustration) to achieve a formulation in terms of a theory of transformations, I arrive at the following: the total analytical experience is being interpreted as belonging to the group of transformations, denoted by the sign T. The experience (thing-in- itself) I denote by sign O. The patient's impression, T (patient) α, is replaced by grid category C2. The patient's representation, a resultant of the transformation he has effected, T (patient) β, is replaced by grid category A1.
>
> (Bion [1965] 2014, p. 138)

> The emotional experience of my illustration, as I have described it verbally, can be represented in the form of an equation as follows: $T = C2 \rightarrow A1$.
>
> (Bion [1965] 2014, p. 138)

Before trying to understand the meaning and scope of this form of representation – in a somewhat esoteric way – it is important to draw attention to some aspects of the passage above. Previously, the *thing-in-itself* was the external fact, the episode of shaking hands, which had already puzzled us. Now, the *thing-in-itself* is the "experience". The mental process of transforming the *thing-in-itself* into a phenomenon – T α – is now referred to as "impression". Now, the term "impression" refers us to an action of the object

DOI: 10.4324/9781003476573-5

on the subject, keeping the subject in the passive (receptive) condition, while T α has suggested an activity so far, a processing engendered by the subject and exercised on the objects. Even in the following sentence, it is clearly stated that the representation results from the transformation the patient "made", emphasizing his activity and, therefore, making the identification of T α with the "impression" even stranger.

We think that many of these landslides could be prevented. Nevertheless, it is necessary and advantageous to arm oneself with a certain tolerance to frustration. Even in the case of seemingly unnecessary shuffling, what stands out is the almost insurmountable difficulty in talking about something that contains an unknowable dimension. It is this unrepresentable dimension – present in all the moments and stages of transformations – that requires a relative colloquial overcoming. In the excerpt above, a sentence that has been omitted is worth taking up:

> Since we have not yet come to a decision about the nature of the process of transformation it is convenient to employ a sign showing that the abstraction represented by T is unsaturated.
>
> (Bion [1965] 2014, p. 138)

The true nature of what corresponds to O, the true nature of what corresponds to T α or T β are irresolute. Just so we don't forget it, a form of representation which does not lead to a false impression of knowing what it is may be useful and, on the other hand, some register is necessary, both so that these elements can somehow be kept at our disposal, as well as to use them in registering certain conjunctions and regularities. We may not know what x, y and z are, but it is convenient to acknowledge that x, y and z tend to occur regularly, forming a pattern, etc. Through the identification of conjunctions, *possibilities of meaning* are formed. This term is not adopted by Bion, but we understand that it reflects a decisive moment in clinical practice: the moment when, from chaos, a pattern begins to form, despite remaining open and demanding new elements which, in turn, will never close it definitively. Let us see how Bion delivers this work project:

> By analogy, we, having bound the constantly conjoined elements of the analytic experience by the formulation $T(\xi) = C2 \rightarrow A1$, may now resort to further analytical experience for evidence which will provide us with meaning: in other terms, to saturate the unsaturated element (ξ); or, again, to put it in another way, we hope to find evidence from analysis for a more precise understanding of this particular patient's transformation.
>
> (Bion [1965] 2014, p. 139)

What can be noticed is that the abstract notation, maintaining the non-saturation and, at the same time, allowing the register of elements' conjunctions, opens up to the future, to the search, to the waiting for new elements.

The great risk of using psychoanalytic theories – metapsychological and, even more, psychopathological theories – is that they excessively impregnate the analytical experience with their images, metaphors, and analogies, so that the field becomes totally saturated. This risk is all the greater the more imbued with images is the psychoanalytic theory, such as Melanie Klein's theory, for example. Nonetheless, patterns will not be formed without the elements being minimally named and interpreted, and this requires psychoanalytic theories. Bion's theory of clinical observation seeks to accomplish the feat of using psychoanalytic theories – without which no interpretations would be formed from the associations – for, then, transposing them in the direction of a form of register that is as much disincarnated and non-saturated with images as possible, so that the field of *possibilities of meaning* mentioned above is continually opened or reopened. The placement of clinical "material" in terms of grid categories is not at the service of a conclusive and strict codification, but, on the contrary, at the service of an ongoing research activity; Bion concludes:

> The investigation of this and other analytical experience should in time enable us to see different types of transformation and perhaps to arrive at some classification of the different sets of transformation which together make up the group of transformations.
>
> (Bion [1965] 2014, p. 139)

The expectation is to elaborate, in a more articulated way, what could be the field of *possibilities of meaning* in the psychoanalytic clinic, sufficiently open and unsaturated so that it does not replace the experience of psychoanalysis but promotes and guides it. It would be a way to learn from the past without obstructing the present or filling the future with determined anticipations. What Bion seems to be looking for is to give greater support to the attitude that Freud called *floating attention*.

That – which took up the first three pages of the second chapter of the book *Transformations* – being said, let us move on to what we consider the "second part". Bion begins to introduce the clinical differences between neurotic and psychotic transformations:

> I assume that mental disorders fall into one of two categories, neuroses and psychoses, and ignoring existing criteria used to distinguish one category from the other I shall attempt to distinguish them on the basis of the theory of transformations.
>
> (Bion [1965] 2014, p. 139)

> In practice this means that I shall regard only those aspects of the patient's behaviour which are significant as representing his view of O; I shall understand what he says or does as if it were an artist's painting.
>
> (Bion [1965] 2014, p. 140)

Bion continues:

> From the analytic treatment as a whole I hope to discover from the invariants in this material what O is, what he *does* to transform O (that is to say, the nature of T (patient) α) and, consequently, the nature of T (patient). This last point is the *set* of transformations, in the group of transformations, to which his particular transformation (T (patient)) is to be assigned. As I am concerned with the *nature* (or, in other words, meaning) of these phenomena, my problem is to determine the relationship between three unknowns: T (patient), T (patient) α, and T (patient) β. Only in the last of these have I any *facts* on which to work.
>
> (Bion [1965] 2014, p. 140)

Then Bion introduces some elements of a clinical case. They are biographical details resulting from the summary of a dream reported before a weekend. Thereafter, the associations evoked by the dream are exposed. This set occupies a half-page paragraph. We will not go into the dream's details and associations. What interests us here is to observe how Bion composes the following paragraph:

> I have chosen this illustration because it lends itself easily to interpretation. The reader can see that the stimulus of the week-end break might be the trigger for the dream and its associations. There is no lack of analytic theories that might be appropriate and with the knowledge of the patient I had – he had been in analysis with me for two years – I was able to narrow choice of interpretations to two or three. But even two or three interpretations can be an embarrassment when one only is wanted and that one correct in the context in which it is given. I am therefore ignoring here, and throughout this book, any discussion of psychoanalytic theories. I am however concerned with theories of psychoanalytic observation, and the theory of transformations, the application of which I am here illustrating, is one of them. Can this theory be applied to bridge the gap between psychoanalytic preconceptions, and the facts as they emerge in the session?
>
> (Bion [1965] 2014, p. 141)

Several aspects call our attention in the passage cited. The first is Bion's belief that certain clinical materials bring a pattern in perfect accord with psychoanalytic theories. For this reason, they almost automatically generate in the reader a high propensity to agree with the interpretation to be offered. We do not know how it is for other readers, but the interpretive process was far from self-evident, although it was plausible. The second aspect worth mentioning is the belief that there may be, among the various interpretations evoked by the interaction between the material standards, the psychoanalytic theories and the patient's prior knowledge, one – and only one – that would be the appropriate interpretation (*correct*) in context. Both beliefs seem to reflect an extremely realistic and scientific view of psychoanalysis, which is surprising for an author who alerts us at every step to the dimension of unknowability. Yet, it also reaffirms the hope that the theory of transformations will mediate the psychoanalytic preconceptions and the unpredictable facts of an analysis session.

That said, Bion continues and, as always, oscillates between a postulation of the unknowability of O – the *thing-in-itself*, now called *absolute facts* of the session – and a language that suggests that O already belongs to the field of experiences of a determined subject, making the distinction between O (patient) and O (analyst), and admitting that they are different, although referred to the same session, to the same stimulating situation. If we effectively take O as *thing-in-itself*, we could not say that it is the same, nor that it is different, because we lack criteria suitable for application to something that does not show itself as a phenomenon. The most reasonable, however, would be to suppose that O is "the same origin" for all who participate in the situation and that differences are created from the plane of transformations. However, Bion states that the first question the analyst should ask oneself is:

> The first question is, what is O (patient), or, to express it in more conversational terms, what was the patient talking *about*? One answer is that he was talking about the week-end break.
>
> (Bion [1965] 2014, pp. 141–142)

We believe that this question is reasonable and obvious. The issue is whether the status of O, as *thing-in-itself*, "absolute facts" and unknowable, is compatible with Bion's question asked above. In the sequence, the question and its possible answer are reformulated – once more! – in terms of the theory of transformations:

> O (analyst), the patient's statements, have been transformed by me, my mental processes being represented by T (analyst) α, to form a view, T (analyst) β, from which I deduce that T (patient) = the week-end break. Or rather that I have assumed that a week-end break, O, exists, and that the phenomena associated with O by the patient is something I denote by T (patient).
>
> (Bion [1965] 2014, p. 142)

In this excerpt Bion highlights the fact that, indeed, a difference between O (patient) and O (analyst) can really be proposed if we consider that T β of each will produce O – or will be a strong ingredient of O – for the other to start his own transformations. Then, it resumes the argument about the advantages of a notation system that can be more precise and less laden with meaning. Finally, he gets to the point:

I shall now consider the state of mind in the patient which makes him see the week-end break as he does, that is, the *process* of transformation T (patient) α. By what mental processes does the patient come to experience the week-end break as an object of fear? What, when he contemplates the week-end break, does he see? In other words, what meaning are we to ascribe to T (patient) β? The material should show both what he sees and how he comes to see it as he does, the process of transformation and the product of that process.

(Bion [1965] 2014, p. 142)

In response to these questions, Bion returns to Freud's theory of transference, as stated in *Beyond the Pleasure Principle* (1920), emphasizing the fact that the repetition occurs with an *unwelcome fidelity*, which would justify the term transference:

The feelings and ideas appropriate to infantile sexuality and the Oedipus complex and its off-shoots are *transferred*, with a wholeness and coherence that is characteristic, to the relationship with the analyst. This transformation involves little deformation: the term 'transference', as Freud used it, implies a model of movement of feelings and ideas from one sphere of applicability to another. I propose therefore to describe this set of transformations as 'rigid motions'. The invariance of rigid motion must be contrasted with invariance peculiar to projective transformations.

(Bion [1965] 2014, p. 143)

The return to the notion of invariance calls our attention. There is a neurotic invariance, which is called transference, or rigid motion transformation, and another invariance: that of projective transformation. In both cases, equivalence between forms is assumed, or the term invariance could not be applied.

In the case of transference, presumably, the *unwelcome fidelity* clearly reveals the equivalence between patterns (forms) of child sexuality and the patterns verified in the relationship with the analyst. It is a transformation that involves little deformation. And this, apparently, in two ways: on the one hand, the same pattern of child sexuality can be recognized in the analytical situation. On the other hand, Bion is convinced: the patient's experience and transformations generate easy and convergent interpretations in the analyst and in his readers. Therefore, it is simple to recognize the past in the present, and the same present in the interpretations that trained analysts could offer in the situation. Ultimately – although unreachable – one can imagine a correct and consensual interpretation to be given in cases of transference neurosis. The interpretation would arise from the intersection of different forms, it would be the best expression of the *something* invariant, of that which is repeated with an *unwelcome fidelity*, but now transformed into opportune fidelity. The realistic premises and certain scientificism mentioned above seem to find their justifications in the clinic of neurosis.

It can be considered, then, that resuming the issue of the invariance and invariants forces the return of the assumption of form that was questioned at the beginning of the second chapter. However, this assumption of form, indispensable in certain aspects and, more than that, required to deal with transference neurosis, is an obstacle to understanding the projective transformation.

The difficulties arise when presenting the clinical material of a case that is not one of transference neurosis. Bion begins the next paragraph by providing registered elements of a session with a psychotic patient. It is a sequence of acts and speech reproduced in a reliable manner and, one can even say neurotic, with remarkably boring fidelity. In the conclusion he confesses:

> The short report is verbally nearly correct; yet as I read it again I see it is a misleading record of the experience. I shall therefore make another attempt to describe this fragment of session but without attempting verbal exactitude.
>
> (Bion [1965] 2014, p. 144)

Therefore, in this case, the exact reproduction of the material is misleading. A long report begins in which Bion's transformations take on a wide space. At the end, he concludes:

> It will be observed that this, my second account of the episode, contains a very high proportion of speculation. The speculations depend on my theoretical pre-conceptions. In addition to classical analytical theory I have had in mind Kleinian theories of splitting and projective identification ... I also assumed that experience of hallucinations, as I have described them in my paper, 'On Hallucination', would stand me in good stead. But beyond preserving an awareness of such a background of theory I allowed myself to be as open to clinical impressions as possible.
>
> (Bion [1965] 2014, p. 145)

At this moment, Bion briefly reports what he feels on the purely affective plane while attending to the patient, and also the ideas that affections themselves seem to generate. There is also reference to a *"mass of details"*, which in the text is disorienting, but which in the clinical situation generates an impact, even though it is not perfectly clear how, since it is difficult, or impossible, to fully comprehend it. One may note then, that the good form reproduced – transferred – from the past to the present, and from the present to an interpretation, is lost. To suppose that T (patient) α and T (patient) β are forms or have form, or even that they are deformations, prevents one from coming into contact with the fragmentary and disintegrated character of what the analyst can capture.

This difficulty in capturing can give rise to doubt: does it result from the patient's difficulty to communicate his experience of O, or from an "intention" to hide this experience? In the illustrative example, Bion assumes that communication chaos derives from the chaotic character of experience itself.

In any case, in a situation like this, certain analyst's transformations – interpretations – that convey an excessive idea of coherence and form can be felt, in Bion's words, as *fanciful* – fictitious and imaginative. In some other times, the interpretations may seem loaded with a certain truth or with effectiveness. But that presumed clarity, and the almost consensual character of the interpretations offered in cases of transference neurosis disappear! In the session fragment's actual presentation, given the ineffectiveness of exact reproduction, it was necessary to introduce Bion's personal speculations, which depend on his experience with the patient. Not only would the interpretations of several analysts not coincide, but the report could also be challenged in its supposed "objectivity".

Thereby, what seems to disappear when abdicating the assumption of form – requirement of the material's fragmentary character – is the notion of invariance, without which it is difficult, if not impossible, to measure the adequacy of interpretation, and even of a narrative. It is one thing to look at a landscape and then recognize that different pictures bring it as a theme, despite the different stylistic principles. It is another to try to recognize the equivalence between different forms – different narratives or different interpretations based on diverse theories – and to say that they "correspond" to a bunch of disconnected doodles. However, according to Bion, projective transformations also contain invariances, but to comprehend them, it will be necessary to move forward in the Bionian text.

References

Bion, W.R. ([1965] 2014). Transformations. In: *The Complete Works of W.R. Bion, Vol. V*, ed. C. Mawson. London: Karnac Books, pp. 115–280.

Freud, S. (1920). Beyond the Pleasure Principle. In: *The Standard Edition of the Complete Psychological Works of Sigmund Freud, Vol. XVIII (1920–1922)*, trans. J. Strachey. London: The Hogarth Press and the Institute of Psychoanalysis, pp. 7–64.

Fourth lesson

The processes of transformation

There is some confusion between "α-function" and "transformation α". There is indeed a movement in Bion's elaborations that needs to be closely followed. That the transformation processes are called T α is not surprising, although before, the α-function referred to a transition from the condition of thing itself (β elements) to the condition of primitive thought. All transitions, including evacuation transitions, are now recognized as containing and implying some transformation, for example, transformation in hallucinosis. The sign α now refers to all transformation processes.

There is some confusion between "α-function" and "transformation α". There is indeed a movement in Bion's elaborations that needs to be closely followed. Let us return to a passage already discussed.

That the transformation processes are called T α is not surprising, although before, the α-function referred to a transition from the condition of thing itself (β elements) to the condition of primitive thought. All transitions, including evacuation transitions, are now recognized as containing and implying some transformation, for example, transformation in hallucinosis. The sign α now refers to all transformation processes.

In Chapter 3 of *Learning from Experience*, Bion states:

> *Alpha-function* operates on the sense impressions, whatever they are, and the emotions, whatever they are, of which the patient is aware. In so far as *alpha-function* is successful, *alpha elements* are produced and these elements are suited to storage and the requirements of dream thoughts.
> (Bion [1962] 2014, p. 174, emphasis added)

Therefore, it is correct to interpret the alpha-function as corresponding to the production of elements that can articulate with each other, in the production of dreams, narratives, calculations, that is, elements that can take shape in the constitution of complex phenomena and processes of mental life. Alpha-elements can either be connected or disconnected, in order to generate other figures in other connections with other enchainments.

DOI: 10.4324/9781003476573-6

However, in *Transformations* Bion uses the sign T α to refer to the transformation process, differentiating it from its product T β. To that extent, T α includes the α-function but is not reduced to it. While the α-function generates elements capable of contributing to the creation of forms – dreams, narratives, formulas, etc. – T α also processes in the reverse direction, destroying forms, inverting the α function, shattering and disintegrating. Chaotic "materials" are thus generated. As I said before, in the normal digestive process – and digestion is a strong model in Bionian thought – both formative and disintegrating movements always and simultaneously occur. Metabolism includes disintegration of nutritious elements so that they can be partly converted into ingredients that maintain the body and are partly evacuated. The worse the digestion, the nearer waste materials will be to the ingested ones. These digestions are usually the quickest: it seems that the material is expelled soon after ingestion. According to Bion, the psychism that works like this is totally regulated by the pleasure principle and does not tolerate any pressure. It is the mind functioning as an expulsive muscle. But even in this case, some processing will have already occurred, that is, the waste will never be the thing ingested in its initial and intact form. On the other hand, however great the use, part of the ingested material will be expelled and, in this case, in an unrecognizable way. Anyway, what matters is to recognize that T α both forms and destroys forms.

The formativity of T α can be determined by a repetitive pattern in which different situations seem easily recognizable by the common pattern, by its invariants. This would be the case of rigid motion transformations, that is, of the transferences. We could proceed by saying that releasing the individual from some of these more limiting and restrictive patterns would correspond to treating his neurosis while maintaining the dominance of the formative aspect of T α.

There are cases, however, in which invariants are not detected in the pattern that determines the psychic capacity of formativity, of creation, but, on the contrary, in the dominance of destructive, disintegrating aspects. In such cases, indeed, the assumption of form – embedded in the term "Transformation" – prevents an adequate conception of the process. Even the term "deformation" is not entirely appropriate, as it is much more about destroying forms than deforming them. The so-called "attacks on linking" (Bion 1959), pertaining to the psychotic part of the personality, would be one of the most radical forms of operation of this mode of psychic functioning, in which all formativity is violently combated.

In fact, in the most serious cases, not only forms are attacked, but, even more so, the equipment capable of generating forms. The equivalent would be the attack of digestive processes in which, for example, gastric juice attacks not the food, but the stomach itself. In psychoanalytic clinic, the attack on the "stomach" manifests as an attack on the analyst's alpha function, as well as his reverie, remembering that reverie is a factor of the alpha function (Bion [1962] 2014). In *Cogitations*, Bion describes this process in a refined way:

"[The analyst] must be able to dream the analysis as it is taking place, but of course he must not go to sleep. Freud has described the condition as one of 'free-floating attention'" (Bion [1992] 2014, p. 209).

But, as the patient cannot support the training of the reverie: "The analyst is to be so treated that he cannot stay awake, and so interrupted and importuned that he cannot go to sleep" (p. 210).

It is clear, therefore, that there is a transformation involved in what the patient does to the analyst – to his body and his mind. What he does – Tp α – however, is to destroy the formative (metabolic) capacities of the analyst, as indeed he has already done with his own.[1] It is interesting to note that this destructiveness does not necessarily take the most obvious forms of aggression. The destructiveness is not essentially in the aggressive contents of Tp β, but in the operating mode of Tp α operation.

Finally, we have come to the third chapter. In this, several aspects that have already been focused on before reappear, so we will make a general allusion to then present what is new.

The first aspect: O's status remains dubious. In the first paragraph, already Bion refers to the patient's O as opposed to the analyst's O, suggesting that they are sometimes different and sometimes identical. In these cases, what may differ – what we must suppose to be different – are the Transformations, both in terms of T α processes and in terms of T β products. As long as it is possible to give up the equivalence between O and thing itself – which cannot be referred to this or that subject – it seems logical and comprehensible to understand O as – in Bion's words – the "stimulating experience". Speaking of stimulating and, even more, of experience, O is necessarily being conceived as already included in the field of phenomena. This, however, will not prevent a long reference to Kant later in this chapter:

> When I assigned O to denote the reality, the impressions of which the individual submits to the process T α, I had in mind what Kant describes as the unknowable thing-in-itself.
>
> (Bion [1965] 2014, p. 153)

Even then, the use of the term "impressions" leaves much to be desired in terms of rigor, when it comes to a reference to the thing-in-itself.

The second aspect: the inadequacy of the means. In the second paragraph, Bion refers to the inadequacy of the means used in the previous chapter to transmit the analytical experience with certain patients and, mainly, the difference between the two cases presented, one of neurosis, the other of psychosis. In the following paragraph, what is called into question is the adequacy of psychoanalysis itself for certain patients. Later on, defects, failures, insufficiencies and inadequacies in the approach being developed will be highlighted. These multiple and varied allusions create, in the reader's affective experience, an atmosphere of perplexity and, perhaps, some discouragement in the face of the intractable complexity of the subject, which will demand an increasing complexity in thought and language. Language complexity, however, which at the same time makes reading more arduous, as we can anticipate, remains insufficient to handle the analytical experience.

Let us return to the third paragraph in which Bion tries to convey clinical experience to us with certain severely compromised patients.

> From the first, it was evident that the resources of psychoanalysis might prove inadequate to the demands of such a patient. In terms of time and money alone treatment would be costly. Patience and a capacity for taking risks were also soon seen to be necessary. It was only necessary for the patient to feel that one demand was satisfied for him to make it the prelude for further exactions; this attitude pervaded all aspects of relationship with me and apparently with life at large. Typical of the development of awareness of a situation to a point at which I could venture on a verbal impression of it, was the fact that awareness grew gradually so that it was difficult to say, when an aspect had been clarified, what material, in the immediate circumstances, was sufficient to sustain the burden of interpretation I wished to lay on it. An interpretation therefore appeared to lack the scientific quality that is conferred by supporting evidence ... A series of such doubts sprang naturally from the fact, obvious at the outset, and therefore of slight significance in the immediate analytic setting, that any collaboration, and particularly an analytic one, with such a patient would be unrewarding and even dangerous. Such premonitions have two mainsprings: the first from the analysis itself, which is so transformed that the intention that the analytic association should be healing and rewarding is frustrated by actions intended to wound; the second from perceptions of the patient's material as it coheres to form his representation of O.
>
> (Bion [1965] 2014, pp. 147–148)

So far, we have a highly suggestive account in emotional terms, although with very few "facts". In fact, it is an account of the countertransference experience that conveys to us the discomfort that such a patient can generate in the analyst.

In continuation, however, Bion makes an interesting observation:

> This first transformation is analogous to that of the landscape gardener who works to transform the landscape itself; the second transformation is analogous to that of the painter who transforms the landscape into a painting.
>
> (Bion [1965] 2014, p. 148)

And he adds:

> It is doubtful whether the transformation of the analysis into something
> wounding should be included amongst transformations in the sense in
> which I have used the term so far. The state of mind in which such
> behaviour is dominant may be described as the patient studying the
> interpretations he receives (Taβ). The object of his study is to arrive at
> action by which he may destroy psychoanalysis.
>
> (Bion [1965] 2014, p. 148)

Before we move on, we should consider the difference between what the gardener who acts on the landscape does and the painter who represents it.
Regardless of whether the gardener's action is formative or destructive – as is
the case with this diabolic gardener who embodies the psychotic part of the
personality – it is necessary to expand the concept of "Transformation", to
include in it processes that result in an action on what until now was O: the
origin of the transformations that the painter makes when representing the
landscape in his paintings. What a patient *does* with the analysis, what he
makes of the analysis – the patient's *use* of objects – to Winnicottize the
issue – implies transformations of a different order than those that result in
the content of what he says, and from which we try to approach the O of his
experience. And that is why, returning to the problem of the misleading
character of colloquial expressions, Bion states:

> The danger that the colloquial sense of a 'transformation of the analysis'
> will infect the meaning I wish to reserve for the theory of transformation
> is one against which I wish to guard by using the sign T. The 'transfor-
> mation of the analysis' refers to a change of 'uses' as set out on the hor-
> izontal axis of the Grid.
>
> (Bion [1965] 2014, p. 148)

Bion and Winnicott are as interested in the "contents" of what is said,
including the flaws in these contents (which lend themselves a certain type of
interpretation more typically Freudian), as to the uses of saying and doing,
which provides interpretations of another type and several forms of "hand-
ling". These other interpretations clarify modes and levels of functioning, and
they are themselves modes of analytical action. It is here that the problem of
"functions" appears and the attempt to categorize – for heuristic purposes –
the various functions of speech is justified, through the use of the grid.

Moving forward, we will find Bion's explanation of the assumptions that
must be supported, even in the face of a disconcerting and threatening clinical
experience: the patient is talking about something that "impressed" him, and
that was transformed by him, and that the result of this transformation is
understandable. Ideally, the analyst should keep his mind open yet prepared

by theoretical preconceptions, in a state of floating attention but with some moments in which certain aspects call his attention – selected facts – enabling him to make meaningful connections. These are the uses of the mind that, according to the grid, correspond to C3, C4 and C5 and D3, D4 and D5. These states should only be interrupted at the time of interpretation, but, in fact, they are not easily maintained in the face of the patient's incessant and often successful attacks. It is interesting to note that the effects of these attacks on the analyst are different from what could derive from counter-transference responses. We believe that many analysts, nowadays, would not make this distinction, as it is a field of difficult differentiation.

After that, Bion makes some considerations about the use of the grid, but we will not deal with it at this moment. He then renews the evidences of the method's deficiencies, but ends by saying that he will anticipate what comes next, pointing out the differences between the material of patients A and B – presented in the previous chapter – calling the first one Rigid Transformation and, the second, Projective Transformation. However, in continuity, he begins the next paragraph bringing a third patient who will later be referred to as patient C – "A patient was speaking of problems in his office". This surprising way of introducing certain themes or materials, without any prior notice, catches our attention. He had just talked about patients A and B and said that from them he would present, in sequence, two types of transformation, but he presents us with a third patient! We shall be patient and lead ourselves despite the fear of being *misled*.

What characterizes the speech of the third patient is the very realistic tone of his report. However, whatever Bion said seemed to have the ability to *lead thinking away*, causing the patient to lose the thread. Coherence was lost, showing how fragile it was: they were split pieces (badly) linked. Any interruption compromised the whole, and any attempt to draw attention to a possible relationship between parts of speech was in vain, as the patient no longer remembered what he had said at the beginning. The interpretation was meaningless. Bion interpreted the situation in Kleinian terms: from schizo-paranoid attacks to the potency of the object with the consequent repercussions on the splittings of the ego. This interpretation had effects on the patient's mood and associations, and thus seemed to be confirmed. At that moment, in the following paragraph, Bion states that hostility appeared less in the communicated subject than in the mode of functioning, and only after this mode was considered, could the contents of the communication make sense.

Well, this third patient is of the type in which the analytical association is frustrating and dangerous. The work slides in an almost uncontrollable way towards the destruction of psychoanalysis, the discredit of the method, the analyst etc. In short: this is what Bion calls "… 'chronic' murder of patient and analyst, or, an instance of parasitism …" (Bion [1965] 2014, p. 28). The patient sucks the resources (knowledge and power) from the analyst, the family, the support groups and all his hosts to strengthen himself and poison them, destroying the conditions for his own existence. How to make this analytical understanding of such a devastating mode of functioning – a mode of *using* an object – possible to the patient's comprehension?

In the following paragraphs, Bion considers some methodological issues and also investigates what would be a prior definition of the stimulating situation of the analyst (Oa), and of the patient (Op). We are concerned with is to know that even if we circumscribe Oa and Op to truly "shared" aspects of the session, this is far from guaranteeing the identity between each other. Patients vary widely in what they include in O.

> In the group of projective transformations, events far removed from any relationship to the analyst are actually regarded as aspects of the analyst's personality.
>
> (Bion [1965] 2014, p. 152)

The example is that of a patient whose "relations" with the milkman or with a boy who whistles on the street, directly affect the figure of the analyst. This is not a transference process, although, to a certain extent, it can be interpreted in this way. If it were transference, it would be a matter of dislocating to the milkman and the whistling boy – affects that concern the analyst – based on the transport (rigid motion transformation) of affects from an archaic source, and according to the infantile pattern. This belief in the dissemination of the transferential relationship, a situation in which many figures in the patient's world are used as support for affects that need to be interpreted by the analyst and aimed at his person, has been part of the Kleinian clinic since the 1930s and 1940s. In these cases, the analyst calls to himself the weight of transferences as if he were always the target, even knowing that on another level he is never the target, even though it may seem to him that the issue is related to himself.

But Bion is talking about something else! He is talking about a state of mind in which the patient does not really know how to distinguish the analyst from the milkman, and thinks – even if he does not say it – that if the analyst does not assume what the milkman has done, it is because he is crazy or acting in bad faith. In this case, the analyst knows almost nothing about O, about what the patient is talking about, because Op includes much more than what could be identified as belonging to the analytical relationship. It is not a matter of reacting to a new object, the analyst, as if it were the old one, one of the parents, for example – transference case – in such a way that both become equivalent in affective terms, which suggests the idea of an invariant form (pattern). In the case of projective transformation, there is a "scatter" of affection that does not circumscribe objects, does not delimit situations, making the recognition of Op an almost impossible task. The limitation or constitution of objects presupposes a certain dominance of the formative and integrating forces of T, and what seems to happen in patients B and C is, in fact, an incessant struggle against forms and formativity itself. To that extent, analyst, milkman and whistling boy, get confused without forming an any more integrated figure.

In the case of rigid motion transformation, the equivalence between archaic and current forms – these being accessible to the analyst who participates in them – one can infer Op as the one that remains, a source of the invariants of transferential relations. In the case of projective transformations, in the absence of these formal invariants recognizable by the analyst, how to look for Op?

Note

1 The similarity between what Bion describes and what was called "attack on reserves" in "Presença, implicação e reserva" (Figueiredo and Coelho Jr., 2008) and "A clínica borderline" (Figueiredo, 2003a) is clear.

References

Bion, W.R. (1959). Attacks on Linking. *The International Journal of Psychoanalysis*, 40: 308–315.

Bion, W.R. ([1962] 2014). Learning from Experience. In: *The Complete Works of W.R. Bion, Vol. IV*, ed. C. Mawson. London: Karnac Books, pp. 247–365.

Bion, W.R. ([1965] 2014). Transformations. In: *The Complete Works of W.R. Bion, Vol. V*, ed. C. Mawson. London: Karnac Books, pp. 115–280.

Bion, W.R. ([1992] 2014). Cogitations. In: *The Complete Works of W.R. Bion, Vol. XI*, ed. C. Mawson. London: Karnac Books, pp. 1–350.

Figueiredo, L.C. (2003a). A clínica borderline [The borderline clinic]. In: *Elementos para a clínica contemporânea [Elements for the Contemporary Clinic]*. São Paulo: Escuta.

Figueiredo, L.C. (2008). Presença, Implicação e Reserva [Presence, Implication and Reservation]. In: L.C. Figueiredo and N. Coelho Jr., *Ética e Técnica em Psicanálise [Ethics and Technique in Psychoanalysis]*, 2nd expanded edition. São Paulo: Escuta.

Fifth lesson

Reading Chapter 3 of *Transformations* (continuation)

Up to the present moment, we have been dealing with the distinction between rigid motion transformations – transference – and projective transformations as ways of differentiating neurotic and psychotic modes of mental functioning. The illustration that refers to projective transformations concerns the patient who is unable to delimit the analyst to configure him as a stimulus to which he responds according to an archaic pattern. The patient in question confuses the analyst with other elements of his experience, such as the milkman or the boy who whistles on the street.

Up to the present moment we have been dealing with the distinction between rigid motion transformations – transference – and projective transformations, as ways of differentiating neurotic and psychotic modes of mental functioning. The illustration that refers to projective transformations concerns the patient who is unable to delimit the analyst, to configure him as a stimulus to which he responds according to an archaic pattern. The patient in question confuses the analyst with other elements of his experience, such as the milkman or the boy who whistles on the street. Let us follow the Bionian text:

> It does not meet the case to suppose that Op, as I am describing it here, is a manifestation of transference, for the term 'transference' should be reserved for the description of the response to a stimulus – whereas I am concerned to delineate the stimulus.
>
> (Bion [1965] 2014, p. 153)

Certainly, not every response to a stimulus is transference, but only when the response repeats an archaic pattern. In order to make the difference between the two forms of transformations, it is necessary: in one case, the existence of a delimited stimulus – the analyst – and in the other, the absence of this delimitation. As mentioned earlier, delimiting stimuli presupposes the preponderance of formative activities. What is assumed in the example given by Bion is that attacks on formativity are predominant, generating states of disintegration, both in the Ego and in its objects.

DOI: 10.4324/9781003476573-7

Both in rigid motion and projective transformations, O, the experience to be transformed – represented – is unknowable. However, in the first case it is possible to achieve a certain notion of what Op would be from the invariants that can be detected in the patient's representations (Tp β) and the analyst's (Ta β). If there is some consensus, a plan of shared knowledge is created – with the help of theory – that is, a common sense of what would be Tp, and from there one can infer what could be Op.

> In rigid motion transformations the invariants establish the relationship with O. But in projective transformations the differences between Op and Oa do not permit of a process of arguing back from Tp and Ta β to Op and Oa as can be done in rigid motion transformations. The crux lies in the nature of Op in projective transformation.
>
> (Bion [1965] 2014, p. 154)

The analyst assumes that it is a stimulus to which the patient responds and, therefore, could be minimally shared. But this assumption does not seem to match the patient's reality. The solution proposed by Bion is to suggest that, in these cases, Op is not a stimulus in the conventional sense of the term, but something that can also trigger a transformation process without the mediation of the perceptible and recognizable stimulus – even if misinterpreted – as occurs in transference. It would then be an element of psychic reality that, in itself, generates a transformation: "A feeling of dread might be such an internal psychic reality" ([1965] 2014, p. 32). What the patient does and says, in this situation, would correspond to a need to represent intolerable affection, projecting it into the elements of his experience, without the contours and limits of these elements being recognized and respected. It is a primitive and radical way of communicating an affective-emotional experience; in Bion's terms: that of projective identification.

In the next paragraph, Bion returns to the example of the painter and proposes a criterion to differentiate between what would be a correct, mediocre painting, and what would be a great painting. In both cases there are formal equivalences – invariants – between the landscape and the painting. In the second case, however, in addition to the correspondence between formal elements – of both terms related – there is an emotional communication by the painter that succeeds in transmitting to those who will contemplate his work, something of his affections when seeing the landscape and composing his painting.

The analyst's situation is somewhat different and partly resembles that of the painter. At first, he will try to help the patient transform the part of his emotional experience of which he is unconscious, to give him a representation; the symbolization effort that allows the patient to acquire his own knowledge. However, when the psychoanalyst seeks to communicate his experiences to colleagues and students, he must proceed as the painter of the "great painting":

The artist is used here as a model intended to indicate that the criteria for a psychoanalytic paper are that it should stimulate in the reader the emotional experience that the writer intends, that its power to stimulate should be durable, and that the emotional experience thus stimulated should be an accurate representation of the psychoanalytic experience (Oa) that stimulated the writer in the first place.

(Bion [1965] 2014, p. 154)

Next, Bion points out the variety of parallels that exist between the painter – but only that of the great painting that evokes emotions, and not that of a mere reproduction – and the psychoanalyst who writes. From these parallels, Bion extracts a new dimension of Transformations:

We may regard the transformation as extending beyond the limits I have imposed if we consider the progression from O to T β as a link in the progression from O to the emotional state stimulated by T β in the observer of the painting, or the reader of the paper. If the emotion stimulated in the recipient of the communication is a *representation* of the emotion stimulated by O in the artist we may regard the artist's intervention in the chain of events as one that does not stop at the disposal of patterns of pigment on canvas, but extends to the emotional state evoked in the individual, or group, and to giving durability to the power to evoke emotion.

(Bion [1965] 2014, p. 155)

And also:

Our model serves psychoanalytic needs better if T β denotes the emotional state stimulated in the recipient and T represents the emotional state, stimulated in the analyst by O, which Ta α is to transform.

(Bion [1965] 2014, p. 155)

Two questions deserve comment. First, the very extension of the concept of "transformation": by placing the emotional effects of T β – whether those of Tp β on the analyst or Ta β on the patient – in the chain of transformations, Bion is already anticipating what he will deal with later on transformations in O. Secondly, by suggesting that emotions are representations of other emotions, and that they are thus representations of O, he is opening up a field of communication for our consideration which is extremely broad and rich, but also disconcerting! For example, if the affections evoked in the analyst (Oa) are to some extent *representations* of the patient's affections which are, in turn, *representations* of Op, it is possible to consider that there is a communication from unknowable to unknowable or – to use the Freudian expression – communication between the unconscious. Therefore, there is excess of communication and, simultaneously, a deficit of communication: much more affection is communicated than the capacities of symbolization available to the analyst (Ta α). Although this paradoxical condition is much clearer when faced with a psychotic or borderline patient – when communication seems to predominantly follow the paths or embezzlements of projective identification – what Bion seems to assume is that something like this is happening universally and, even more, that this is part of normality and health. The inability to use projective identification communication is, in itself, a sign of serious impairment of psychic functions.

In the next paragraph, Bion ([1965] 2014, p. 155) emphasizes O's unknowable character and adds the fact that patient and analyst can only have their feelings, their emotional experience, to have some idea of what is going on between them and with them. The "material" available for access – strictly forbidden – to Op and Oa is that of the patient's and analyst's verbalizations, and the emotional states generated by words. Bion wonders about the status of the verbalizations and the affections they generate, in terms of being T β with greater or lesser propriety, and also of *being* or merely *representing* an emotional experience. However, he seems to conclude that these questions are not essential, although they stem from the painter's model, which, by giving rise to certain questions, may prove to be *misleading*. He then says, harping on the same string of the inadequacy of symbols in face of the demands of symbolization: "I shall retain both model and signs until something better becomes possible" (Bion [1965] 2014, p. 156).

Following the text, Bion ([1965] 2014, p. 156) starts the paragraph somewhat unexpectedly. Addressing the reader directly, he tries to confront an emotional reaction that his book may be generating: what psychoanalysis book is this, in which there is no talk of sexuality, anguish, conflict, Oedipus? He then finds himself obliged to repeat and clarify that his book is not related to the main body of psychoanalytic theory, but to the practice of psychoanalytic *observation* – and the term observation is set in italics. However, what would appear to be a self-imposed restriction on his elaborations is revealed in another way:

> Psychoanalytic theories, patient's or analyst's statements are representations of an emotional experience. If we can understand the process of representation it helps us to understand the representation and what is being represented.
>
> (Bion [1965] 2014, p. 156)

To understand the speeches of patients or analysts as *representations of affects* – more than, or as much as, descriptions of well-perceived stimuli – is presumable. However, as if passing by and without any fuss, psychoanalytic theories are also brought to the field of transformations. It is not just a matter of understanding them as instruments capable of detecting and promoting the emergence of patterns in the patient's "material"; they would be – in themselves – representations of emotional experience. In taking this idea to its ultimate consequences, one must admit that psychoanalytic theories contain, in themselves, the disproportion between excess and lack, that is, they contain an emotional effectiveness – an ability to generate emotional states – greater than their own capacity to symbolize them. There is a tendency, in theories, to privilege only their instrumental dimension. What Bion allows, however, is for the recognition of another dimension in them: as representation of O, the term "representation" not being reduced to the field of ideas. Theories will never fully know what they are dealing with, and what they theorize about. Going further, there would be an efficacy of theories that is difficult to understand or control, that is, the capacity of theories to produce emotional states through a primitive form of communication. This could also be used to explain the "preference" for this or that school of psychoanalytic thought or, on the contrary, the antipathy that certain texts and styles generate in certain readers.

Let us return to the text:

> T β may be expressed through the medium of speech. Psycho-analysts agree that correct analysis demands that the analyst's interpretation should formulate what the patient's behaviour reveals; conversely, that the analyst's judgment should be embodied in an interpretation and not in an emotional discharge (e.g. counter-transference or acting out). To this we may add provisionally that his contribution may be regarded as embodied in the change in the patient's emotional state.
>
> (Bion [1965] 2014, p. 155, p. 156)

> T β may be expressed through the medium of speech. Psychoanalysts agree that correct analysis demands that the analyst's interpretation should formulate what the patient's behaviour reveals; conversely, that the analyst's judgement should be embodied in an interpretation and not in an emotional discharge (e.g. counter-transference or acting out). To this we may add provisionally that his contribution may be regarded as embodied in the change in the patient's emotional state.
>
> (Bion [1965] 2014, p. 156)

It is expected that the emotional experiences produced in the analyst by the patient will be sufficiently elaborated to emerge as spoken interpretations, and not as discharges. For this to occur, they must be incorporated into the process of change and the patient's affective states to be effectively "good" interpretations. This will require the analyst to continuously monitor the patient's emotional state. It is to facilitate this task that Bion uses the "grid". Through the grid, he tries to identify the nature of the elements the patient uses to represent his emotional experience, and the precise uses he makes of these elements.

The content of the communication, so important in analysis, will be touched on only incidentally in the discussion of transformations; it will depend on O as deduced from the material in the light of the psychoanalyst's theoretical pre-conceptions.

(Bion [1965] 2014, p. 157)

As already noted above, no matter how decisive the contents are, they are not everything, nor the most important. Bion emphasizes the resources, uses and modes of mental functioning as ways to identify patients' emotional states and their transformation strategies. In the following paragraph, Bion ([1965] 2014, p. 157) suggests, the theory of transformations, although it seems to concern psychotic personalities, must be understood in a more general plan. This is due to the importance given to projective transformations, more evident in psychotic personalities, since in rigid motion transformations all the work of deductive access to O is facilitated. That leads to the mistaken impression that the theory of transformations is more about psychotic personalities.

Before concluding the chapter, Bion ([1965] 2014, p. 157) repeats the warning against the limitations of the painter's model: *misleading*, but still useful! He then refers to the text "Formulations on the Two Principles of Mental Functioning" (Freud, 1911); in which Freud distinguishes two modes of functioning. In the first one, muscular action occurs to alter the environment immediately; in the second, the thinking is interposed. Bion suggests that many phantasies are considered "actions" capable of discharging excess stimuli from the mind. It would be the case of Kleinian projective identifications through which affections – which are intolerable representations of an O condition – need to be evacuated in order to generate an equivalent representation in the recipient. Mental development presupposes this ability to communicate through projective identifications. Let us go to the text:

The growth of insight depends, at its inception, on undisturbed functioning of projective identification. If it is disturbed, mental development is hampered by the phantasy that insight depends on what is regarded, even by the sophisticated mind, as action.

(Bion [1965] 2014, p. 158)

The disruption of projective identification would correspond to a breakdown in the early stages of mental development, in the capacity for insight – to make contact with the emotional experience through the mediation of another continent that is capable of reverie. The result, paradoxically, would be the preponderance – throughout life – of this mechanism of communication with the other, which is, at the same time, an avoidance of communication with oneself. However, it would always appear in an exaggerated, hyperbolic, and highly destructive way.[1] The β elements – non-metabolized affections – would constantly exert on the patient's protomental apparatus – a true evacuation muscle – a terrible pressure, requiring discharge through action. These would be the projective transformations in their specific difference in relation to rigid motion transformations, the transferences.

Note

1 In Attacks on Linking, Bion (1959), develops his argument on the consequences arising from the impossibility of resorting to splits and projective identifications in their normal and healthy forms.

References

Bion, W.R. (1959). Attacks on Linking. *The International Journal of Psychoanalysis*, 40: 308–315.

Bion, W.R. ([1965] 2014). Transformations. In: *The Complete Works of W.R. Bion, Vol. V*, ed. C. Mawson. London: Karnac Books, pp. 115–280.

Freud, S. (1911). Formulations on the Two Principles of Mental Functioning. In: *The Standard Edition of the Complete Psychological Works of Sigmund Freud, Vol. XII (1911–1913)*, trans. J. Strachey. London: The Hogarth Press and the Institute of Psychoanalysis, pp. 218–226.

Sixth lesson

Reading Chapter 10 of *Transformations*

After going through the first three chapters of *Transformations*, we propose a jump to the last three since the aim is not to accompany the entire work of the author but to exercise the capacity for deconstructive psychoanalytic reading. In Bion, as mentioned at the beginning, the focus – to be permanently unfocused and refocused – falls on the status of O. Therefore, we will use Chapter 10, presented as a review and summary of the book but which reveals itself as going beyond that.

After going through the first three chapters of *Transformations*, we propose a jump to the last three, since the aim is not to accompany the entire work of the author, but to exercise the capacity for deconstructive psychoanalytic reading. In Bion, as mentioned at the beginning, the focus – to be permanently unfocused and refocused – falls on the status of O. Therefore, we will use Chapter 10, presented as a review and summary of the book but which reveals itself as going beyond that!

Bion begins by proposing another model of transformation, leaving behind that of the landscape painter. It is a game with marbles, of different colours and sizes – ½", ¾", and 1" in diameter – arranged on a tray. Suppose a rule: on another tray, as many marbles of 1" in diameter are placed as there are green marbles on the first. After performing the entire operation, the marbles on the second board will represent an aspect of the arrangement of the marbles on the first. Let us call the first tray O; the rules will correspond to T α and the marbles on the second board will be T β. On the other hand, those marbles on the second tray will be the O of a next transformation, and Bion will represent this equality through an equation: O (2nd cycle) = T β (1st cycle). In other words, the equivalence between the result of a transformation and the condition of the unknowable as the origin of a next transformation is well established here.

Now suppose another rule: on a third tray, as many marbles of 2½" in diameter will be placed as there are blue marbles on the second. This would be a rule of type Tα (2nd cycle) that would generate a new T β (2nd cycle) that would be like O (3rd cycle) for the resulting transformations. Imagine that the relations between the arrangement of the marbles – on the first and

DOI: 10.4324/9781003476573-8

third trays – are far from obvious, and with each new tray the apparent equivalence becomes more tenuous and more difficult to detect. However, each of the boards would be assembled according to very precise rules and would represent an aspect in the formal arrangement of the marbles on the previous tray. Each is the previous one, now transformed, but the possibility of recognition between the different trays and the O of the 1st cycle becomes progressively more precarious.

This leads us to an infinite process of distance and deviation, in which very simple and determined rules of transformation operate. Bion will try to bring the example of the trays to something closer to the analytical experience. A paragraph will then begin, and we should follow it:

> ... suppose the patient makes a complex statement, in the sense I have given the term, which may have consisted of anything from a solitary ejaculation to a session of free associations. I shall suppose that the statement is so complex that it would only be adequately represented by being categorized in every grid category. The categories, like the sizes and colours of the marbles, may be regarded as 'dimensions' of the statement.
> (Bion [1965] 2014, pp. 240–241)

This multidimensionality requires that one or a few dimensions are – at each time – selected to give way to a Ta β interpretation. The complete statement will be for the analyst O (1st cycle), corresponding to the first tray with marbles. The Ta α rule will be equivalent to the choice of a given dimension to generate Ta β, the interpretation. What can one think of the analytical activity, applying to this second model what we have already learned from the first, the one of marbles on the different trays?

Note that the second transformation model proposed by Bion as a paradigm of the psychoanalytical process is precisely that of the succeeding trays with marbles. Again, each of the trays is assembled according to a rule that defines a dimension of the previous tray and, from there, represents this base-tray by arranging the balls on the following tray. In the sequence, each tray is a transformation very much determined by the previous one. Each transformation, in turn, will be the source of the next one. However, despite this well-established chain, the relationship between the last transformations and the original tray is almost undetectable.

Bion suggests that the patient's material, in particular his speeches, can be taken as the original tray – O – endowed with enormous complexity, in the sense that it contains elements from all categories of the grid. Exposed to this material, the analyst is led to select a certain dimension, from which he constructs his interpretation. Such an interpretation would therefore be a transformation of O from a certain angle, which includes the selected dimension and the theoretically established transformation rule.

The transformation of O [patient's speeches, therefore Tp β] into Ta β [an interpretation made by the analyst] is associated with K link, assuming that the transformations of O (original patient experience) into Tp β are associated, mainly to L, H and -K, although one must also assume a participation of K. This means, in everyday words, that the patient is moved by love (L), hate (H) and refusal of the truth (-K), even if a part of him is looking for it. The analyst's transformation is predominantly at the service of truth, of knowledge. Hence, we could say that the transition from O (to the analyst, they are the patient's transformations driven by love, hate and refusal of the truth) to Ta β (an interpretation) corresponds to transforming an emotional experience into knowledge. However, this knowledge conveyed to the patient will inevitably be transformed according to the individual's transformation rules, associated with L and H, and, ultimately, it must return to the status of emotional experience, that is, it must overcome the limits of a knowledge level and return to the condition of O. For this to occur, however, the force of -K must be attenuated.

What Bion wishes to emphasize is the impossibility of knowing with certainty something about the rules that generate these sequences of transformations: "The conclusion must be that we must make assumptions about assumptions about ... *ad infinitum*. No conclusion is possible about the arbitrary nature of the rule" (Bion [1965] 2014, p. 242). However, in the analyst's case, the rule can be seen as a case of preconception, an idea or theoretical psychoanalytic model that operates in the analyst's observations, organizing and directing his attention, preparing him for certain phenomena, waiting for "filling". Bion says:

> Ta α is a private process limited to the analyst's mind: the categorization of Ta α impinges on the domain of counter-transference and the analyst's own analysis. The matter is relevant to discussion of the nature of the relationship of interpretations to the matter interpreted. The assumption underlying loyalty to the K link is that the personality of analyst and analysand can survive the loss of its protective coat of lies, subterfuge, evasion and hallucination and may even be fortified and enriched by the loss. It is an assumption strongly disputed by the psychotic, and *a fortiori* by the group which relies on psychotic mechanisms for its coherence and sense of well-being.
>
> (Bion [1965] 2014, p. 242)

This paragraph brings together two important themes. First, the relationship between the analyst's transformation processes and his emotional experiences evoked by contact with the patient and his material. The selection of a dimension of the material and the use of a "rule", an idea or a theoretical model depend on something that goes beyond cognition.

What characterizes the analyst's position and his activity is his *loyalty to the K link* and his conviction that he and the analysand will survive the truth and both will become stronger with it, this being the second aspect. Bion has no doubts: *what heals is the truth*, although it is not the truth in the most conventional and purely intellectual sense of the term. It is the animistic capacity to welcome, get in touch with, recognize, and name the emotional experiences.

The healing by truth opposes the powerful forces of the psychotic mechanisms that operate in all individuals and, mainly, in groups. These only remain united and happy through resorting to psychotic mechanisms, that is, by the use of very intense manifestations of the L and H links, primitive expressions and communications of indomitable and unsymbolizable love and hate. From this view of the groups as inevitably committed to the most primitive forms of communication and to non-thinking, one can draw both a quite negative critique of the collectivities and, on the contrary, a more tolerant view in the face of madness ("Without madness, what is man ..."? Fernando Pessoa). What would an unlimited capacity to think thoughts lead us to? Would not there also be, in this extreme lucidity, a very pernicious form of madness?

Continuing, Bion suggests that when interpreting a material, the analyst should consider exclusively the elements that can be categorized as β elements being evacuated (A6), that is, as actions of expulsion of the non-symbolized elements. It is not necessary to always do this in analytical practice, but the situations in which this selection imposes itself are the most complex and difficult in conducting a healing process. These situations are those in which words are said yet often devoid of their symbolic function; they are words used as ejectable things, that is, used with an evacuation function. We would be mistaken if we tried to understand what is happening in terms of effective symbolic communication, both considering the patients' speech and their listening and reaction to the analyst's interpretations. We can assume that even in patients whose quality and use of psychic elements are more sophisticated, many lines need to be taken as expelling actions of β elements. That is, even though they "communicate", they are behaving as "non-communicating" when using words that are no longer in the place of the non-object (an absence that propitiates thought), being themselves the presence of an object that blocks the space of thought.

One can say that the equation is simple, or relatively simple: thinking is only done in the absence of the object; whereas the absence of the object is frustrating, and the frustration is painful. If one cannot bear the psychic pain of frustration, there is no room for thought; if there is no space for thinking, one cannot build a thinking apparatus, and if there is no apparatus for thinking, the absence of the object and the pain of frustration are intolerable. If, in turn, these experiences are intolerable, they must be expelled. In general, these expulsive movements generate pernicious effects in the "outside world", but if someone can receive these toxic projectiles as primitive forms of

communication – although they are nothing more than evacuations – to welcome, contain, transform etc., only then to return them at the right time and
in the right measure, an apparatus for thinking can gradually be built. However, there will always be leftovers of proto-thoughts – waste that is almost
mental and almost corporeal – to be disseminated around the world in search
of an unrelated, collective and impersonal apparatus for thinking.

Bion makes the equivalence between the words spoken and the air expelled
from the lungs, so that the brain becomes, in this case, an organ of excretion.
Not only the "talking" brain, but the sense organs themselves start to behave
as parts of a digestive system and, more than that, of a very primitive and
even defective digestive system: what goes in, goes out, and must go out even
by the routes that are usually entrance, as in vomiting. The mouth behaves
like an anus, and the same can happen with the eyes and ears that hallucinate.
Instead of being entrances, hallucinating eyes and ears are exits through
which unbearable emotions are expelled; they gain, in hallucinations, figur-
ability in the "external" world, but mainly, they conquer a supposed "externality" when evacuated. In this figurative externality, apparently signified,
while relieving the patient, even being terrifying hallucinations, they affect the
analyst, who should not confuse them with proper symbolic communications.
But what to do with them, how to interpret them? After a quick illustration
of how he was affected and was able to deal interpretatively with evacuations
of this order – projective transformations of the patient – Bion recognizes:

> My account of these events cannot be made plausible to anyone who has
> not had the analyst's experience. I shall not attempt to make the
> description convincing but shall pass on to consider implications of this
> and similar ineffable experiences.
>
> (Bion [1965] 2014, p. 244)

In other words, even if we share with the analyst his preconceptions – psychoanalytical ideas and models – we have no way of sharing his clinical
experiences, much less his experience with this patient. To this extent, the
analyst's O and the transformation rules that operate in him are inaccessible
to us; hence, his account will seem arbitrary and unconvincing. The "original tray" with its marbles and the rules for composing representations of
this O tray are not within the reach of an external observer and, most likely,
neither are they completely clear to the analyst himself – who is affected and
interprets them as if they were communications – which results from evacuations vaguely addressed to the "outside". These evacuations may either
come in the more or less undisguised form of β elements (disjointed phrases,
screams, faces, gestures and other bodily manifestations, etc.), or they may
be primitive uses of more sophisticated elements. The grid, while distin-
guishing the quality of the element from its use, allows several nuances to be
discriminated.

Following the text, Bion states his conclusions in synthetic form of small paragraphs, numbered from 1 to 6. It will be convenient to follow him step by step:

1. Hallucination is seen as a method of achieving independence which the patient considers to be superior to psychoanalysis (Bion [1965] 2014, p. 245).

By making the sense organs function "in reverse", expelling affections and generating figures, the individual not only relieves himself of tension through the evacuation route, but also fills the absence of the object with his own resources, becoming imaginarily autonomous and self-sufficient. When this mechanism is dominant, the patient assumes that his method of dealing with frustration is much better than that proposed by the analyst, who imposes, in a certain way, the experience of frustration.

2. Its failure, in so far as it is seen as a failure, is attributed to the rivalry, envy and thieving propensities of the analyst (Bion [1965] 2014, p. 245).

The impossibility of making hallucination a perfect method – especially when in analysis the patient is confronted by the analyst – is interpreted by the analysand under the dominance of the H link, as if a much better method than psychoanalysis resulted from the analyst's hatred. It would be interesting to consider how certain "therapeutic" or "analytical" interventions can corroborate, or can give effective support, to these delusional interpretations; the fight against resistance and, even more, the patient's claim to self-sufficiency and arrogance are effectively capable of generating a countertransferential hatred that cannot be concealed.

3. Rivalry, envy, greed, thieving, together with his sense of being blameless, deserve consideration as invariants under hallucinosis (Bion [1965] 2014, p. 245).

In addition to rigid motion transformation (transference) and projective transformation, already contemplated in this path, Bion also considers the transformation in hallucinosis. In it, O – the emotional experience – not only produces evacuating and relieving movements, but generates figures that, imaginatively, fills the lack of the object and completely avoids the experience of frustration and pain. Bion suggests that inevitably this omnipotent method of self-healing is associated with feelings of rivalry and envy that are projected on the analyst.

4. The concept of hallucinosis needs to be widened to fit a number of configurations which are at present not recognized as being the same (Bion [1965] 2014, p. 245).

There is more hallucination and delirium than it seems at first sight. The expanded concept of hallucinosis includes a transformation rule that can be conceived in more abstract terms and with less obvious detection than the mere presence of the hallucinated object; it is not just a matter of seeing and hearing "ghosts", but of supplying oneself, maintaining omnipotence and self-sufficiency. To this extent, the presence of hallucinosis may be more pervasive than it appears.

5. Transformation, in rigid motion or projection, must be seen to have hallucinosis as one of its media (Bion [1965] 2014, p. 245).

While rigid motion and projective transformations could even articulate in concrete cases, yet without being confused or overlapping, transformation in hallucinosis can be conceived as one of the means of other transformations and not as an independent modality of transformation, although it has its own rules.

6. The rules of transformation in hallucinosis must be established through clinical observation. I have no doubt that they exist and can be delineated by observation of the operation envy, greed, rivalry, "moral" and scientific superiority in hallucinosis. I offer the following suggestions provisionally as an example of such "rules" (Bion [1965] 2014, p. 245).

Before we follow Bion in these suggestions, it is worth emphasizing once again what is decisive in characterizing the transformation in hallucinosis: the combination of an intense affection in the face of idealized alterity (envy, rivalry and voracity) with the pretension of omnipotent self-sufficiency (superiority, arrogance); it is from this explosive combination that some rules of this transformation derive:

a   If an object is "top" it dictates "action"; it is superior in all respects to all other objects, and is self-sufficient and independent of them.
b   Objects that can occupy such a position include (a) Father, (b) Mother, (c) Analyst, (d) Aim, object or ambition, (e) Interpretation, (f) Ideas, whether moral or scientific.
c   The only relationship between two objects is that of superior to inferior.
d   To receive is better than to give (Bion [1965] 2014, p. 245).

As can be seen, these rules of transformation in hallucinosis do not emphasize the production of imaginary figures, but rather ways of interpreting phenomena and relationships, on the one hand, and on the other, postures and attitudes. It is a mode of mental functioning endowed with some invariants, although these are not found primarily – as in the artist's model – in some formal equivalence between the landscape and the painting or – as in rigid motion transformation – between archaic and current situations. However, these invariants have an extraordinary power to generate identity and repetitions that dramatically restrict the variability of the world, reducing it to a single and universal code in which the novelty of a relationship (for example, the novelty of analysis) finds no place. There is a narcissistic encapsulation in the "same", which is always experienced in a binary mode (active x passive, superior x inferior), in which the inferior is subjected (passively) to the obligation to give, and the superior actively imposes the demand to receive. The creation of the hallucination pseudo-object is already an attempt to respond and reverse this situation.

At this moment, Bion introduces a new approach to differentiate rigid motion transformations (transference) and transformations in hallucinosis: a mathematical approach. The mathematics of rigid motion transformation would be:

a^1 The infant feels it is being satisfied by the breast: the breast disappears and the satisfaction with it.

a^2 1 breast + 0 breast = 0 breast
a^3 1 + 0 = 0
 (Bion [1965] 2014, p. 246)

In this case, the child can endure the absence and tolerate some frustration. Suppose, however, that she cannot experience absences, tolerate frustrations and their resulting pain. The math for hallucinosis would be:

b^2 1 breast + 0 breast = 1 breast
b^3 1 + 0 = 1
 (Bion [1965] 2014, p. 246)

The following paragraph needs to be carefully analyzed:

There may be good reasons for supposing that $1 + 0 = 1$, for example that there is a realization that may approximate to it, and the formulation $1 + 0 = 1$ may help to establish a K link with such a realization. But b^3 is intended to demonstrate the relationship between 0 and 1 in a domain where it is possible to remove the 'noughtness' from 0 and so produce 1. Therefore, in the domain of hallucinosis $0 - 0 = 1$. It is natural to wonder what would be the result of adding nought to nought. It is $0 + 0 = 0°$. That is to say that if noughtness is added to noughtness, the noughtness is multiplied by itself. The emotional state that might provide a background realization approximating to this is the state of complete freedom from the restriction imposed by contact with realizations of any kind. The ability of 0 to increase thus by parthogenesis corresponds to the characteristics of greed which is also able to grow and flourish exceedingly by supplying itself with unrestricted supplies of nothing.

(Bion [1965] 2014, pp. 246–247)

The consideration of this passage requires us to face the translation of *noughtness*.[1] *Nought* can be translated as *nothing*. However, *nought* is a direct reference to the digit 0 (zero). Tic-Tac-Toe (or noughts and crosses), in which, obviously, 0 corresponds to a sign like any other. The winner is who gets a row of three crosses or three zeros, in this game, it means $0 + 0 + 0 = 3$. To take *noughtness* from 0 is to treat 0 as thing (or name of thing) and not as nothing, nothingness, absence. In this case, nought becomes 1 (one digit).

The mathematics $0 + 0 = 0°$, however, which describes the case of hallucinosis, shows that in addition to taking *noughtness* out of *nought* (taking nothingness from 0, leaving a unit in place), this transformation makes the absence – contained in the noughtness of nought – self-inseminating. Instead of the absence giving way to frustration, it generates itself, enhanced, in the form of an insatiable and growing voracity, feeding on "unlimited supplies of nothing".

That said, let us go back to the passage mentioned above. Accepting that $1 + 0 = 0$ implies a well installed capacity to accept the nothingness of zero, to accept the loss of the breast, of satisfaction, to accept the irreparable loss of unity and completeness. It will be in the presence of $1 + 0 = 0$ (in remembrance of an irretrievably lost satisfaction) that, in the place of the no-thing, thought may emerge. On the other hand, supposing that $1 + 0 = 1$ could still be justified by the hope that some realization may re-edit the old satisfaction of the encounter with the breast. In this case, $1 + 0 = 1$ would prepare the subject for this re-encounter (for example, in the form of an ideal), even if the re-encounter would never occur.

However, in the transformation in hallucinosis, the first step was to remove nothingness from 0, refuse the absence and transform the sign of absence into a form of presence. Therefore, $0 - 0 = 1$, putting in words, zero devoid of zeroness is equal to 1 digit. In addition, the sum of absences (noughtness added to noughtness) generates an unrestricted voracity. What is refused is pure and simple absence, which leads to pure and simple frustration. On the one hand, the absence is cancelled by the presence of the sign-thing 0, on the other, and, at the same time, voracity is increased exponentially by the supplies of nothing that feed it.

The combination of these two aspects of the transformation in hallucinosis determines what we could call death of desire. In its place, zero devoid of zeroness manifests itself as hostile envy and voracity. Contrary to the frustrating absence, more accepted and that sustains desire, hostile envy and insatiable voracity *are in themselves the presences that fill the lacks*, emotional states that occupy and invade the individual with, or even, without the explicit hallucinating images. Under the mathematics in which $1 + 0 = 1$ and $0 + 0$

$= 0°$, everything is full and excessive, and the individual feeds on himself, therefore, always being excessively filled.

Considering that the transformation in hallucinosis is one of the means of rigid motion transformation (neurosis) and projective transformation (psychosis), and considering that the psychotic and non-psychotic parts of the personality are, according to Bion, present and active in each of us, it is understandable that the concept of hallucinosis should be extended, and that psychoanalytic treatment should be able to deal with this mechanism as one of its main therapeutic tasks.

The task is to embed absences at the fulfilling breast. This is much more difficult than it seems because every experience of absence will be, under the logic of hallucinosis logic, an opportunity for fulfilment and excess. Therefore, it is not enough to be absent, silent, to abstain, to frustrate, to play dead, to make cuts and other fine mottoes. The math of $0–0 = 1$, $1 + 0 = 1$ and $0 + 0 = 0°$ transforms all these magnificent strokes of absence into full unwavering presences!

Note

1 T.N.: the passage is kept close to the original, favoring the etymological discussion.

Reference

Bion, W.R. ([1965] 2014). Transformations. In: *The Complete Works of W.R. Bion, Vol. V*, ed. C. Mawson. London: Karnac Books, pp. 115–280.

Chapter 7

Seventh lesson

Continuing reading Chapter 10 and starting Chapter 11 of *Transformations*

In the tenth chapter of *Transformations*, presented at the beginning as a "review and summary", we have found, so far, a large number of new ideas that go way beyond what could be a synthesis of what has already been presented. In the first place, the transformation model of the painter who reproduces a landscape is replaced by that of the tray with marbles of different diameters and colours, which is transformed into other trays – according to very well-determined rules – apparently disconnected from the initial, but which, in fact, represent it according to colour and size dimensions established by each transformation rule. This novelty, transposed to the psychoanalytic relationship, does not summarize but expands the possibilities of thinking about what goes on between analyst and analysand in terms of sequences of quite complex and not very obvious transformations. But the great novelty of this chapter is in the postulation of a mode of transformation – transformation in hallucinosis – that may be present in neurosis, although it is more active in psychosis, and which, therefore, is articulated with rigid motion transformations (transference) and projective transformations.

In the tenth chapter of *Transformations*, presented at the beginning as a "review and summary", we have found so far, a large number of new ideas that go way beyond what could be a synthesis of what has already been presented.

In the first place, the transformation model of the painter who reproduces a landscape is replaced by that of the tray with marbles of different diameters and colours which is transformed into other trays – according to very well determined rules – apparently disconnected from the initial, but which, in fact, represent it according to colour and size dimensions established by each transformation rule. This novelty, transposed to the psychoanalytic relationship, does not summarize, but expands the possibilities of thinking about what goes on between analyst and analysand in terms of sequences of quite complex and not very obvious transformations.

But the great novelty of this chapter is in the postulation of a mode of transformation – transformation in hallucinosis – that may be present in neurosis, although it is more active in psychosis, and which, therefore, is

DOI: 10.4324/9781003476573-9

articulated with rigid motion transformations (transference) and projective transformations.

In the presentation of the transformation in hallucinosis, Bion introduces an odd mathematics in order to show how absences, lacks and nullities (noughtness) can be abolished and filled by something that the subject himself generates from the frustration and other affections that the absences produce in him. Everything that could be empty and the absence of an object – the condition for the production of thoughts and for the constitution of a thinking apparatus – is immediately transformed into a hallucinated plenitude, even if no hallucinations are produced in the strict sense of the word.

Accompanying Bion along the trails of this surprising mathematics, we understand that there is a basic opposition between, on the one hand, the acceptance of frustration – the ability to experience the voids – and, on the other, hallucinosis. To focus on the realization that corresponds to the acceptance of frustration, Bion ([1965] 2014, p. 247) writes: 1 breast + 0 breast + 1 breast + 0 breast + 1 breast + 0 breast + 1 breast + 0 breast = - 4 breasts. This means that when there is an ability to accept the absence, the sum of alternating experiences of satisfaction and frustration expands the space of tolerable lack. When, however, frustration is impossible – when the transformation in hallucinosis predominates – 1 breast + 0 breast = "one breast denuded of existence" and "a place where the breast was, yet also denuded of existence" = "a raging inferno of greedy non-existence". Voracious non-existence is the nothing that fills and feeds itself.

In the expanded space of absence, instituted by the alternation of satisfaction and frustration, when there is a possibility to accept frustration, the possibility of *knowing what a breast is* opens up, even though this determination sends us to an unknown dimension of reality (to be researched). In the case of hallucinosis, on the contrary, there is no room for any knowledge, for any transformation according to rules that apply to definable dimensions of reality.

In the next paragraph, Bion ([1965] 2014, pp. 247–248) introduces an idea that will only be developed further below. It is a matter of questioning the current notion of psychoanalytic interpretation as having the purpose of turning the unconscious into conscious. It already seems that the thought of transformations establishes greater possibilities by inserting psychoanalytic interpretation into a complex sequence of transformations that, according to the grid, admits much finer categorizations than that provided by the binary distinction between conscious and unconscious. In addition, interpretations must be understood in the context of the psychoanalytic relationship.

In the case of the patient who resorts to transformations in hallucinosis, the analyst's interpretations will inevitably be inserted in the context of a rivalry between the two methods for dealing with suffering. The psychoanalytic method seeks to expand the spaces of tolerable void, the tolerance to frustration; the patient's self-healing method here characterized as transformation in hallucinosis, on the contrary, tries to abolish the experience of frustration.

What is more complicated is that the failures of this second method – because it inevitably fails in reality-check – will be attributed to the analyst's envious attacks. The more accurate his interpretations, the more apt, in principle, to install spaces of absence, and greater the chances of being heard as attacks on the patient's ability to self-sufficiency through the use of hallucinosis in which he creates his own objects of fulfilment and satisfaction.

Then there is a short paragraph in which Bion ([1965] 2014, p. 249) differentiates hallucination from what would be an illusion: he speaks of illusion or delusion; in Portuguese it is difficult to find two terms that contrast in a corresponding way to English terms. Delusion, however, can be understood as a mistake, a mistaken belief, differing slightly from what is an illusion. In this case, the translation of delusion by "delirium" does not seem to me to be good for strengthening the distinction intended by Bion. Illusions or mistakes, in a few words, can be corrected because they refer to a reality that is not self-produced. Illusions are preconceptions that require saturation and that are not an evacuation of senses. Hallucinations, on the contrary, do not refer to anything but themselves, they are their own saturation and only marginally come into conflict with something that can deny them – hunger only, which persists despite the baby eagerly sucking what serves as a soother, denies the effectiveness of the breast hallucination.

Hallucinations and, in general, transformations in hallucinosis, express narcissistic omnipotence and, to this extent, imply, by their very nature, a rivalry: they are means by which the subject asserts his self-sufficiency and his superiority before the whole "not me" reality. The baby who falls asleep smiling and sucking the thumb on which the mother's hallucinated breasts presents itself, will be saying: "I'm the one!" It is in this context that a psychoanalytic interpretation can effectively ruin the hallucinated bliss. Finally, in the face of hallucination, two vertices must be considered: that of the patient and that of the analyst. What for the analyst is hallucination, for the patient is the reality made to his measure and built entirely with his own resources.

To speak of these two vertices, however, Bion introduces a digression that will come to have a very broad scope in the continuity of his work, and in another thematic context. He will resort to Plato's theory of forms:

> As I understand the term, various phenomena, such as the appearance of a beautiful object, are significant not because they are beautiful or good but because they serve to 'remind' the beholder of the beauty or the good which was once, but no longer is, known.
>
> (Bion [1965] 2014, p. 250)

The next step is to bring the theory of forms and knowledge as a reminder of Plato, of his own theory of preconceptions and innate object anticipations. To this extent, although the phenomena that form the basis of the representations are transformations of O, "… the significance of O derives from and inheres in the Platonic Form" (Bion [1965] 2014, p. 250).

This Platonizing step establishes, in any case, one of the poles in the understanding of O. O is inaccessible to the senses and, in itself, does not phenomenalize. However, it would already contain in itself the matrices of possible phenomena. These become recognizable when they remind us of something that, curiously, can never be known directly. This is a relationship of knowledge, within the limits of the possible.

Before going any further, it is worth noting that this way of conceiving O as already endowed with an organization – a transcendental order, sustained in Platonic forms – puts O in a quite different position from what Bion has told us so far and will say, even more radically, later. If O carries this transcendental order, it may be inaccessible to the senses, but it is not at all unknowable, since it would open up itself to the knowledge of O, the vast field of reason. As will be seen later, O, far from having well-defined forms, is postulated as a formless void, from which forms can be "extracted" in a process of "achievement", in which the phenomena are constituted. The hypothesis that the phenomena are merely imperfect replicas of the transcendental forms does not seem very appropriate to the unknowable character of O, although it can be effectively approximated to the innatism of inherited preconceptions.

Bion is still interested in the Christian modality of Platonism and, in this case, the phenomena are not a memory of forms, but an incarnation of the person of God that allows the subject to meet with God through his incarnations. In this case, we go beyond a relationship of knowledge, as the meeting takes place as participation and communion. It is much more letting oneself be inhabited by the divinity, through contact with its incarnation, than to know it, indirectly, through the phenomena that remind us of transcendental forms. The mystical experience will be, as we shall see, a model for this modality of transformation that is no longer a transformation of O, but a transformation into O, it is no longer a knowledge of O, but being (becoming) O.

Where can one go via this unexpected route through Platonism and Christianity? It seems that Bion is trying to present us, analogically, what can be conceived about the "relationships" with O from two different vertices. On the one hand, it is really about *relations*: Love, Hate and, mainly, Knowledge (the analyst's vertex). Loving, hating or knowing are ways of linking to the original experience (O) and, to this extent, generate transformations of O that can themselves be objects of love, hate and knowledge. In a way, we could say that L, H and K are always inadequate for O, although they are appropriate for transformations of O. In each of these links there is a kind of exaggeration and detachment, which is at the root of what Bion calls hyperbole. Not only all love and hate, but all knowledge, even that considered "objective", precisely because of this is hyperbolic and differs from being O. In the same way, *acting out* (the field of performance) is different from *acting* (the field of taking action).

Before concluding Chapter 10, which unfolds and contorts over its many pages (it is one of the largest in the book), Bion ([1965] 2014, p. 253) discusses the dynamics of hyperbole as a means of – through exaggeration – clarifying and drawing attention to certain aspects of reality. In hyperbole, the embossments of reality are accentuated, and in some way they can impose themselves ("hollering"), although other aspects are attenuated or eliminated by hyperbolic deformations. There is, therefore, a loss of O. Then Bion returns to the matter of the psychoanalytic relationship with the patient who resorts do hallucinosis in an accentuated way, either because of innate characteristics or by the intensity of early relationships.

Although we could continue meditating on Chapter 10, the digression that remained partially in the air – on Platonism and Christianity and on the vertices – takes us directly to Chapter 11in which the question of "relationships with O" is much more elaborate.

> My theory would seem to imply a gap between phenomena and the thing-in-itself; all that I have said is not incompatible with Plato, Kant, Berkeley, Freud and Klein, to name a few, who show the extent to which they believe that a curtain of illusion separates us from reality. Some consciously believe the curtain of illusion to be a protection against truth which is essential to the survival of humanity; the remainder of us believe it unconsciously, but no less tenaciously for that.
>
> (Bion [1965] 2014, p. 258)

The curious list draws attention at the beginning, both by the names included and by the ones left out. It is remarkable the height and vastness in which Bion places his thoughts and themes, in the field of epistemology and, even more widely, of existence.

Bion says that even those who believe that the truth should be attained, usually admit that we are not cognitively prepared for it. However, "From this conviction of the inaccessibility of absolute reality the mystics must be exempted" (Bion [1965] 2014, p. 258). On the other hand, and as a result, the mystic's great difficulty in communicating emerges, since all the means of ordinary language are capable to deal with phenomena and their transformations. Although Bion is not presenting himself as a mystic, he does not fail to remind us that for him, too, the search for suitable forms of expression is as necessary as it inevitably fails. Like the mystic, the psychoanalyst has an experience of O that can neither be disqualified nor transformed into adequate representation, since every transformation of O is somehow hyperbolic.

Much of Chapter 11 deals with the limits of knowledge as access to O and, at the same time, as an eventual propitiator of a transition to O, of a transformation in O, of becoming O.

The gap between reality and the personality, or, as I prefer to call it, the inaccessibility of O, is an aspect of life with which analysts are familiar under the guise of resistance. Resistance is only manifest when the threat is contact with what is believed to be real; there is no resistance to anything believed to be false. Resistance operates because it is feared that the reality of the object is imminent; O represents this dimension of anything whatever – its reality.

(Bion [1965] 2014, pp. 258–259)

The first noteworthy aspect – which will be emphasized by Bion later on – is the anti-processual character of *resistance*: resistance is triggered by the *imminence* of the "reality of the object" and breaks out to face it. In turn, O is this very imminence, that is to say, this dimension of reality as what is to come. It is the transition to O that is prevented, much more than the knowledge of O. The knowledge of O can even be one of the ways of not passing to O, of preventing its imminence. What is at stake is not knowledge and its vicissitudes, that is, man's cognitive capacities and limits, but the frightening possibility of passing to O, of becoming O; on the verge of O. Following Bion:

To recapitulate: It is possible through phenomena to be reminded of the 'form'. It is possible through 'incarnation' to be united with a part, the incarnate part, of the Godhead. It is possible through hyperbole for the individual to deal with the real individual. Is it possible through psychoanalytic interpretation to effect a transition from knowing the phenomena of the real self to being the real self?

(Bion [1965] 2014, p. 259)

The issue, therefore, concerns psychoanalytic efficacy and not just the "truths" of psychoanalytic knowledge. After this problematization, Bion returns to the question of the purpose of interpretation in psychoanalysis, left in the air in the previous chapter:

If I am right in suggesting that phenomena are known but reality is 'become', the interpretation must do more than increase knowledge.

(Bion [1965] 2014, p. 259)

However, to what extent does this concern the analyst? Would not this step be, necessarily, that of the patient, or at least of that part of the patient capable of making contact with O? Before answering the questions, Bion makes room for an important distinction: in making contact with O, two very different positions can be taken. One is to suppose God, to embody omnipotence, omniscience and to go astray in megalomania. The other is to let oneself be taken and affected by O: "Moreover, health may be more easily associated with being passive, *vis-à-vis* ultimate good and evil, rather than with being active" (Bion [1965] 2014, p. 259). Anyway, having started playing on the team of Plato, Kant etc., it is now time to get off the high horse!

Bion takes up the argument to emphasize the gap between knowing psychoanalysis and being psychoanalyzed, but his objective is to discuss resistance, since it is often situated exactly as an obstacle that prevents the transposition of this gap.

> In terms of resistance theory the aim of resistance is to preserve unconsciousness of thoughts, feelings and 'facts', presumably because that is felt to be the best method, *in the circumstances*, of dealing with the problem presented by those thoughts, feelings and 'facts'. Resistance cannot, however, be evoked unless there is in operation the contrary feeling that consciousness is the best approach.
>
> (Bion [1965] 2014, p. 260)

There are several aspects to be highlighted. First, the heterogeneity of the elements of O that may, in their imminence, trigger resistance movements: thoughts, feelings (affections) and "facts". We must assume that these different dimensions of O require different defence mechanisms. In particular, resistance to "facts" suggests that there is a mechanism capable of counteracting facts in their imminence, that is, a defence mechanism against contact with reality that is more radical than those responsible for preserving the state of unconsciousness of thoughts and feelings.[1]

A second aspect is Bion's emphasis of the tense and conflicting character that the term "resistance" contains: there is resistance only when there is, in the opposite direction, pressure towards truth, towards reality. It is the imminence of O, as a feeling that accepting and welcoming O may be the best solution – albeit a painful one – that unleashes resistance to O. In fact, both pressures on which resistance acts are confused. Resisting the truth, on the one hand, frees the subject from many pains; on the other, it can burden him excessively.

It can often be more practical and simple to oppose the coming (or returning) of thoughts, feelings or "facts". Our daily life, "normal" daily life, is full of episodes of this type of resistance in which the imminence of O occurs without major problems. However, a pathological situation sets in when the encounter with O must be avoided and postponed infinitely. In this avoidance and in this postponement, we are dealing only with transformations of O. This means that not only when the H (Hate) link prevails, but also when L (Love) and K (Knowledge) prevail – situations in which O is only hyperbolically present – there is always a resistance to O (in its imminence) operating. Letting oneself do O, becoming O, overcoming resistance to the imminent O is something that psychoanalyst Ignácio Gerber, using Zen terminology, would characterize as *detachment*, and which we consider one of the main forms of *reserve*.

In the continuation of Chapter 11, the ideas about the transformation in O and the resistances to this movement of becoming – as opposed to knowing – are not developed immediately. The question that seems to move Bion's thoughts at this moment is how transformations of O should be conceived in essence and, in the answer to this question, a certain understanding of O takes shape, distinctly from the one in which O was supposed, preordained according to the transcendental forms *à la* Plato.

The argument goes, first, by the notion of number. Numbers are the most abstract devices to gather elements that appear in regular constellations; they, in a way, identify and cut out regularities (constant conjunctions), making them available for further research and understanding. However:

> Psychologically the problem commences with the impingement on the individual of an object containing in itself the potentiality of all distinctions as yet undeveloped …
>
> (Bion [1965] 2014, p. 261)

It is through the *impingement* of O on the individual that the possibility is created, and even the necessity of establishing cuts and gathering of elements, that is to say, it is in this invasive impact of O that certain possibilities of uniformity are generated, this happening from an *object* that holds the *potentiality of all distinctions as yet undeveloped*. Therefore, they are not eternal and finished forms waiting to be remembered from contact with phenomena. This nature of O becomes even more evident when Bion uses a verse by Milton in *Paradise Lost*: "The rising world of waters dark and deep / Won from the void and formless infinite".[2]

The rising world of waters dark and deep – does not have any of the good delimitation and intelligibility that one would expect from the phenomena – it is won from this even more indeterminate plane, which is the *void and formless infinite*.

We have, therefore, three conceptions of O. In the first, O is preordained by the Platonic forms that are recalled by contact with phenomena that, in turn, become recognizable when they evoke the memories of eternal forms. If O were like this, resistance would hardly be understood as resistance to the transition to O. On the other hand, it helps to understand what innate preconceptions would be, the inherited tendencies to organize the world according to certain patterns.

In the second conception, O does not contain fully constituted Platonic forms, but a *potentiality* for all distinctions not yet developed. In this version, the reason for resistance is still very poorly understood. Why, after all, would it be so frightening to come into contact with the "object" imposed on the individual, already suggesting certain lines of ordering? On the other hand, this version suits Bion insofar as it supports the thesis in which the contact with the experience triggers, enables and demands recognition and construction of patterns that make the material more comprehensible – a material which, for its part, already contains these patterns as possibilities.

It is worth noting that in these two versions there can be no attempt to bring O closer to the Kantian thing-in-itself since, in Kant's terms, the patterns according to which the phenomenal world is organized are conditioned by the subject – the transcendental subject – and not by more or less determined aspects of the object. That is why the list of authors that Bion identifies with is so strange, and begins by associating Kant with Plato and Berkeley.

Finally, we have the idea of O as *void and formless infinite* – a *nothing of entities*, in Heideggerian terms – from which the world emerges in a still chaotic state. In this case, it is much easier to identify the reasons for resistance. What generates resistance is the anguish in the face of the *void and formless infinite – nothing* of entities – and, probably, the dread of the emerging world of *dark and deep waters*, because the world here is not acquired, from *nothing*, in the form of something simple and well discriminated. In this version, the status of O as unknowable finds its full formulation. In this case, however, all the reasoning about constant conjunctions, regularities, from which we could start making sense of things by organizing them into phenomena, remains unsupported.

However, it is from this last conception of O that Bion concludes that knowledge – K – involves the process of binding through which the representable entities are formed.

> The process of binding is a part of the procedure by which something is 'won from the void and formless infinite'; it is K and must be distinguished from the process by which O is 'become'.
>
> (Bion [1965] 2014, p. 262)

If we considered K, in some way, as derived from the incipient forms of O that falls on the subject, this transformation of O would be part of becoming O. However, placed in confrontation with the void and formless infinite, K differs from becoming O and, to a certain extent, needs to be understood as part of the resistance to O – the nothing of entities – in its imminence. Hence the question: can we, from this plan of transformation of O, which is the psychoanalytic knowledge, the psychoanalytic interpretation, provide a transformation in O?

Notes

1 A discussion of *Verleugnung* in these terms was developed by Luís Cláudio Figueiredo in the text "*Verleugnung*. A desautorização do processo perceptivo", in *Elementos para a clínica contemporânea* (São Paulo: Escuta, 2003).
2 John Milton, *Paradise Lost*, Bk. III, 1667.

References

Bion, W.R. ([1965] 2014). Transformations. In: *The Complete Works of W.R. Bion, Vol. V*, ed. C. Mawson. London: Karnac Books, pp. 115–280.

Figueiredo, L.C. (2003). *Verleugnung*. A desautorização do processo perceptivo [*Verleugnung*: The disauthorization of the perceptual process]. In: *Elementos para a clínica contemporânea* [*Elements for the Contemporary Clinic*]. São Paulo: Escuta.

Chapter 8

Eighth lesson

Reading Chapter 11 (continuation)

Continuing his considerations about K and its limits, Bion points out that the notion of causality belongs to this plane, to the transformations of the O plane, according to K. Although one cannot contest the legitimacy of the uses of the notion of causality, "The interpretation should be such that the transition from knowing about reality to becoming real ..." (Bion [1965] 2014, p. 153). The conditions for this to happen do not allow themselves to be thought according to a simple notion of causality, and they issue a radical challenge to our capacity for expression and understanding. We are here, indeed, in one of the most substantial and most decisive nuclei of Bionian thought and difficult to penetrate.

Let us go back to Milton: "The rising world of waters dark and deep / Won from the void and formless infinite".[1]

Bion, after the transcription, warns:

> I am not interpreting what Milton says but using it to represent O. The process of binding is a part of the procedure by which something is "won from the void and formless infinite"; it is K and must be distinguished from the process by which O is 'become'. The sense of inside and outside, internal and external objects, introjection and projection, container and contained, all are associated with K.
>
> (Bion [1965] 2014, p. 262)

Let us highlight the following aspects:

1 One of the indispensable representations of O, but not the only one, is the one suggested by Milton, who, as we have seen, presents chaos – *the void and formless infinite*, the *nothingness of entities* – as the "source" from which something can be constituted;

2 In this process of becoming, the emerging world, acquired from the "formless", is far from showing clarity and distinction: it is a world of dark and deep waters and, perhaps for this reason, only a poet can offer us a representation of O and the emerging world;

DOI: 10.4324/9781003476573-10

3   In any case, this representation, like any other, is not a becoming O; it is a knowledge operation (K link) that acts through links, creating figures and groups of figures from gathered elements;

4   What may go unnoticed, however, is the scope of the last sentence in which Bion affirms that inside and outside, internal and external are associated with K link. *Binding*, maintaining the meaning of "linking", includes others. For example, the term bookbinding, in a sense of covering the book, protecting it, delimiting its outline. In other words, the operation of binding is also an operation of bringing together and enveloping, setting limits. Bion aligns a series of oppositions that, in the Kleinian and Bionian tradition, refer to primitive and universal processes, to say that all are associated with K and not with O. K generates transformations of O and is appropriate to these transformations, but is not suitable for O. For O, "inside" and "outside" do not apply, nor do all the other oppositions that derive from it. With this, he accentuates the insurmountable gap between the logic that governs the world of concepts – even if these concepts aim at the unknowable – and the void and formless infinite plane in which the experience is born.

Continuing his considerations about K and its limits, Bion points out that the notion of causality belongs to this plane, to the transformations of O plane, according to K. Although one cannot contest the legitimacy of the uses of the notion of causality, "The interpretation should be such that the transition from *knowing about reality* to *becoming real* …" (Bion [1965] 2014, p. 153).

The conditions for this to happen do not allow themselves to be thought according to a simple notion of causality, and they issue a radical challenge to our capacity for expression and understanding. We are here, certainly, in one of the strongest and most decisive nuclei of Bionian thought and it is difficult to penetrate. Says Bion:

> This transition depends on matching the analysand's statement with an interpretation which is such that the circular argument remains circular but has an adequate diameter.
>
> (Bion [1965] 2014, p. 263)

To further specify this notion of "adequate diameter", he says that if the diameter is too small, it becomes a point and, if it is too wide, a straight line, and that both alternatives correspond to primitive states of mind and not to mature experiences. Bion continues:

> The profitable circular argument depends on a sufficiency of experience to provide an orbit in which to circulate. To re-state this in terms of greater sophistication, the analytic experience must consist of knowing and being successively many elementary statements, discerning their orbital or

circular or spherical relationship and establishing the statements which are complementary. The interpretations that effect the transition from knowing about O to becoming O are those establishing complementarity: all others are concerned with establishing the material through which the argument circulates.

(Bion [1965] 2014, p. 263)

In order to understand – although not completely – what Bion tells us, we must start by focusing on *matching* the statements of analysand and analyst. Requiring an interpretation to *match* the statements of the analysand suggests, firstly, that the interpretation neither adds nor subtracts, although it differentiates. It is not a mere repetition as such, but neither is it a causalistic explanation. In *matching* there is a come-to-meet in the form of some equivalence. However, this *return to the saying* that is a *return of the saying* – hence the notion of "circularity" – must be able to circulate through a field. A field that is neither too open (the straight line that would be the correlate of a very wide diameter, that loses contact and distances itself) nor too closed (the point that does not circulate and is repeated), that is, it must have the adequate diameter. Sometimes, an interpretation must incorporate elements to escape the force of attraction of the point that repeats. At other times, it must be able to interrupt a drift in order to circumscribe a field in which the return is possible. In one way or another he seeks to allow the saying to come to itself in its own scope, the appropriate diameter through which the experience circulates.

Throughout the analytical experience process, this *matching* provided by the return to / of the saying through a circulation, according to an appropriate diameter, leads to a succession of *knowing oneself* and *becoming* many of the elementary statements, discerning their relations and establishing their complementarities and correspondences.

It is worth highlighting the distinction proposed by Bion between mutative interpretations (he does not use this term) that favour the transition between K and O, and other interpretations that establish *the material through which the argument circulates* (Bion [1965] 2014, p. 263). This second one, it seems, is exclusively committed to K link, although they prepare the occurrence of the transition from K to O.

Bion postulates a certain equivalence between the transition from K to O and the transition from a preconception to a conception (Bion [1963] 2014). The important thing about this approach is the idea that a preconception that is realized – which is saturated by the encounter of what realizes it, turning into a conception – can retain its capacity to function as a preconception, open and waiting for new realizations. This is what happens repeatedly throughout the scientific research process. Hence, Bion can state: "The psychoanalytic conception of cure should include the idea of a transformation whereby an element is saturated and thereby made ready for further saturation" (Bion [1965] 2014, p. 264).

This little repair is interesting because when we talk about the transition from knowing to being we could convey the idea that *becoming* O would mean a fulfilment, a realization that would saturate and "satisfy" a certain "hunger to be". For Bion it is important to emphasize that the transformation in O, at the same time that it realizes, it also maintains the openness and availability for new saturations. It could not be otherwise, since the transformation in O corresponds to a certain return to the void and formless infinite, in which the limits have not yet been set. There is, therefore, on one hand, a radical opposition between the transformation in O and the transformation of O into hallucinosis, in which faults and frustrations are abolished. On the other hand, there is a certain similarity between the transformation in O and the transformations in O governed by K link, at its most developed levels. The research work, for example, is not yet becoming O, but it does not structurally oppose this transition, since in both cases the lack of saturation (the non-filling of the voids) is important. Likewise, a certain type of mystical experience is not yet the transition to O, but it is similar to it in the possibility of remaining close to the void and formless infinite as well as to the dark and deep waters.

In order to conclude the reading of Chapter 11, we focus on the last paragraph in which Bion takes up the topics we are dealing with:

> To rigid motion transformations, projective transformations, and transformations in hallucinosis, I shall now add transformations in O. That is to say I propose to extend the significance O to cover the domain of reality and 'becoming'. Transformations in O contrast with other transformations in that the former are related to growth in becoming, and the latter to growth in 'knowing about' growth; they resemble each other in that 'growth' is common to both.
>
> Transformation in K has, contrary to the common view, been less adequately expressed by mathematical formulation than by religious formulations. Both are defective when required to express growth, and therefore transformation, in O. Even so, religious formulations come nearer to meeting the requirements of transformations in O than mathematical formulations.
>
> (Bion [1965] 2014, p. 266)

I will point out next five aspects: first, the obvious opposition between the neurotic and psychotic transformations and the transformations in O. Second, the extension of the significance of O; it is not just a matter of understanding O as *reality* in itself and unknowable, but of introducing O into the temporal dimension of *becoming*. We had already referred to this when speaking of O in its imminence. O is inseparable from the movement of becoming, and this is why the resistance to O is, ultimately, resistance to time. In a passage from this chapter, Bion says:

> In thinking about transformation we may arrest the process, at whatever point we wish, to give ourselves the conditions in which to make our inspection. If carried to extremes the process of arrest can amount to a denial of the passage of time ...
>
> (Bion [1965] 2014, p. 262)

Although the research activity (K) requires the interruption of the continuous process of transformations, when taken to extremes, what is configured is a resistance to O in the form of denial of time.

Third, in an unannounced way, Bion introduces the contrast between transformations in O and transformations of O governed by K link. The expression growth in becoming seems to demand, as a "translation", something in terms of an expansion in the capacity to accept O in its imminence, that is, growth of the psychic capacity to be, understanding this "being" not as a substantive state (a substance), but as a potentiality and, to this extent, as a verb.

The fourth aspect is that "growth in becoming" contrasts with "growth of the knowledge about growth", but in both cases the notion of growth appears. It is a very awkward notion (like so many others used by Bion, such as "personality", "maturity" etc.) to the epistemologically educated ear. However, what is important in this notion of "growth" is, first of all, a reference to the process of expanding a certain psychic capacity, and second, it is about expanding the capacity to accept what goes beyond what has already been lived, felt or known. Opening spaces, or keeping spaces open for the experience with everything that it contains of void and formless infinite is proper to both the *growth in becoming* and the growth of the capacity to think.

The fifth and last aspect consists of the following: although scientific and mathematical transformations, as well as the religious ones (in fact, these are attempts to express mystical experiences) fall short of the question of transformations in O, both are close to it, the religious ones being nearer to becoming O than the mathematical ones. This theme will be taken up in the next and last chapter of the book *Transformations*, but we can already anticipate that the relative privilege of religious transformations seems to lie in the fact that mystics accept more easily than scientists the unknowable character of O, the void and formless infinite.

After having marked these five aspects, we shall move on to the last chapter (Chapter 12) of *Transformations*.

The chapter begins with a controversy between Berkeley (philosopher and bishop) and Newton regarding differential calculus. We are not interested in differential calculus itself, nor in Berkeley's critique of what is specific to this scientific device. What results from Bion's use of this episode, however, is relevant. Fundamentally, the issue is that in the transformation of O, governed by K link, there is always something that must be avoided in the experience of the object under examination. In the experience there are aspects capable of generating psychic "turbulence" that compromises the field of knowledge, and that will participate in knowledge in a spectral form, a ghost. In the case of differential calculus, the flows themselves (the movements) that are the *raison d'être* of the calculation should be kept out of the calculation as "spectra of quantities already gone". In much more general terms, what emerges is the idea that knowing implies the ability to evade contact with the aspects of the object of knowledge that generate turbulences which are correlative to a transformation in O.

However, the march of transformation in K may be obstructed when it approaches dangerously what could be a transformation in O. It is not the fear of knowledge itself that generates resistance, but the fear that K will transit into O causing what Bion refers as psychic turbulence. This turbulence is elucidated resorting to St John of the Cross and notions of "dark nights of the soul".

In Bion's interpretation, the first "dark night" that the soul must endure to enter into mystical contact with God corresponds to the pains involved in the realization of the "naivety" state, inseparable from connection or definition operations. In order to create connections, it is necessary to support ignorance, the absence of objects and figures already formed. It is what Bion calls "admission of the negative dimension" and what we can refer to in terms detachment or reserve. Detachment or reserve are conditions for accepting the turbulent potential of the void and formless infinite and, even more, of the emerging world of dark and deep waters. In the impossibility of tolerating this darkness, there tends to be a rush towards objects such as they are, which characterizes the transformation into hypochondriasis.[2]

Likewise, the intuitive approach is obstructed because "faith" – the surrender to the object involved in contact with O – is associated with the absence of rational research, that is, with the suspension of conceptual cognitive operations.

Finally, the third "dark night" is directly associated with the transformation in O, the transition from K to O. What Bion claims is that this transition always carries with it the risk of the unlimited and the fear of megalomania of one believing that is God, almighty and omniscient. While the first "dark nights" refer to states of deprivation (seeing nothing, understanding nothing), the third threatens with an excess.

It is not difficult to understand the fact that the interpretations can also be used as resistance and obstacles to the transition from K to O. Interpretations, especially those easily accepted by the analysand, can serve for a kind of collusion in which the pair can simultaneously conserve the K link and interrupt the transition to O. Bion says that these interpretations are maintained as elements of Column 2 – the column in which all the elements that, regardless of their level of elaboration, are used to fill the faults and interrupt the processes of elaboration – in order to prevent, finally, access to the truth.[3] An interpretation thus used functions as a saturated concept that prevents the K → O transformation, imprisoning analyst and analysand in the field of a supposed knowledge.

Notes

1 John Milton, *Paradise Lost*, Bk. III, 1667.
2 Bion talks about Transformation in hypochondriasis and not hypochondria. The Brazilian translation for "Transformação em hipocondria" [Transformation in hypochondria] does not seem to be adequate. We do not have more precise information, but we think that the relationship between hypochondriasis and hypochondria is equivalent to that of hallucinosis and hallucination. We consider that a transformation into hypochondriasis corresponds to a way to sensorialize a turbulence that is generated in a non-sensorial plane, the plane of the dark night of the senses; the individual projects turbulence into the sensory body.
3 This column refers to a use that Bion calls ψ.

References

Bion, W.R. ([1963] 2014). Elements of Psycho-Analysis. In: *The Complete Works of W. R. Bion, Vol. V*, ed. C. Mawson. London: Karnac Books, pp. 1–86.

Bion, W.R. ([1965] 2014). Transformations. In: *The Complete Works of W.R. Bion, Vol. V*, ed. C. Mawson. London: Karnac Books, pp. 115–280.

Chapter 9

Ninth lesson

Reading Chapter 12 of *Transformations*

Our main objective is to investigate the status (or statuses) of O. For this reason, we will take another leap in the Bionian text, to appreciate a paragraph that offers a contribution in the desired direction. The theme covered in this excerpt refers to the relationship between the theories of psychoanalysis – on which Bion does not intend to operate, but on which he depends – and what he is building in *Transformations*: a theory of observation.

Our main objective is to investigate the status (or statuses) of O. For this reason, we will take another leap in the Bionian text, to appreciate a paragraph that offers a contribution in the desired direction. The theme covered in this excerpt refers to the relationship between the theories of psychoanalysis – on which Bion does not intend to operate, but on which he depends – and what he is building in *Transformations*: a theory of observation. Theories of psychoanalysis and the theory of observation overlap:

> The domains of Theories of Observation and Theories of Psychoanalysis overlap, but the problem is simplified if a distinction is made and can be preserved.
>
> (Bion [1965] 2014, p. 270)

The example that is to come, which is not in itself a clarification, but suggests a solution, is the following:

> 'Hyperbole' is the term I give, in theories of observation, to the realizations that correspond to the theory of projective identification.
>
> (Bion [1965] 2014, p. 270)

The same phenomenon or process can be understood as "projective identification" and as "hyperbole". What is gained and what is lost in each of these ways of thinking? What is gained from the overlap? And, simultaneously, with the distinction between these codes?

Theories of psychoanalysis capture their objects in relations with the mental apparatus, its history (real or assumed) and its mechanisms. The

DOI: 10.4324/9781003476573-11

theory of observation covered by Bion tries to capture them in their relations with the analyst in the *here* and *now* of a session. Bion understood that psychoanalytic theories "applied" directly to the clinic would lose their unsaturated character, that is, they would pre-empt the field of investigation. This is what often tends to occur in the Kleinian clinic. An observation theory has the function of conserving the space of research and singular experience. On the other hand, theories of observation become sterile without the broader and deeper perspectives that psychoanalytic theories offer. It is necessary, therefore, that they overlap, without being confused, that is, that the analyst always has this *binocular vision*, being able to look at the same target from two vertices, from two codes. If we remember that for Bion there is no perfectly adequate representation of O, the possibility of having (at least) two angles of view, two interpretation codes, prevents a single angle and a single code from being placed as a superior and authentic form of contact with reality. There will always be the possibility and need to work with both and *between them* – as in stereophonic listening – without fixing on a single perception. Considering that a work of psychic elaboration always supposes the ability to address each phenomenon from different angles, getting around and considering it from different places, the simultaneous operation of psychoanalytic theories and the theory of observation contributes to the elaborations of the analyst, freeing him from the enclosure that any angle, even those supposedly privileged, produces. Let us skip, however, the digression on the hyperbole, to resume contact with the text when it revisits the question about O. We will now have to face a long, uphill stretch with dangerous curves:

I shall reconsider O with the help of (ξ), Platonic Forms and their 'reminders' (phenomena); 'godhead', 'god' and 'his' incarnations; Ultimate Reality or Truth and the phenomena which are all that human beings can know of the thing-in-itself: all three possess a similar configuration. Milton can invoke light which at the voice of God invested

> The rising world of waters dark and deep
> Won from the void and formless infinite.

Eckhart considers Godhead to contain all distinctions as yet undeveloped and to be Darkness and Formlessness. It cannot be the object of Knowledge until there flows out from it Trinity and the Trinity can be known. According to Kant the thing-in-itself cannot be known, but secondary and primary qualities can be. Examples of similar configurations can be multiplied, but for my purposes these are sufficient to indicate what I mean to signify by O (without, I hope, distorting the historical meanings that the authors wished to formulate).

According to need it may be supposed that (i) from O undeveloped distinctions evolve, or, that (ii) from O, the "void and formless infinite", the individual (sense) and group (common sense) win secondary and primary qualities (in Kant's sense). The 'winning' of qualities is part of K. In so far as potentialities and distinctions 'evolve' from O, it is a part of becoming or Transformation in O. Transformations in K may be described loosely as akin to 'knowing about' something, whereas Transformations in O are related to becoming or being O, or to being 'become' by O.

(Bion [1965] 2014, p. 272, emphasis added)

At the beginning of the transcribed excerpt, Bion approaches the three conceptions of O: Platonic forms to be remembered in contact with phenomena, divinity as incarnation potential, the ultimate reality of the unknowable thing-in-itself. It is worth pointing out that the first meaning will not return in the following passage. In fact, the Platonization of O seems to be the most paradoxical and unjustified resource in an author who intends to emphasize the unknowable character of the reality of experience.

In the sequence, Milton's verse appears again, and then an allusion to the mystic Master Eckhart. In Eckhart, as read by Bion, there are two notions dear to him: that the divinity itself is darkness and formless, but that already contains a possibility of "evolution" which makes it possible to generate a basic form – the Trinity – through which it can be indirectly known. We will see later how this duplicity is useful for Bion's purposes.

Soon after that, he makes reference to Kant, to the unknowable thing-in-itself and to the known secondary and primary qualities. With these multiple references – which he feared to use improperly, but hoped not to deform too much – Bion hopes to put us on the edge of what he wants to say about O. It is important to note that neither Eckhart, nor Kant, and much less Plato say what Bion wants to say about O, they just place their readers – therefore, us – on the threshold of what Bion will say next. Each of these authors brings us closer to this threshold, preparing us to listen to Bion. Given the absence of adequate representation of O, neither the words of Kant, Plato, Eckhart, nor those of Bion himself will be able to say fully what would be worth saying. But for this very reason the task of saying must walk along these tortuous paths in which we approach a place, bypassing it countless times, almost arriving without arriving, getting nearer yet farther, etc. From each angle you can see a piece, you can never see it straight and completely.

We emphasize "According to need". It is evident that for Bion it is also clear that we cannot approach darkness without the risk of losing it, and that therefore we must, *according to needs*, open alternative and always limited approach paths. Thus, we can assume that O is a field of possibilities for "evolution", in itself inaccessible, but whose "products" can be known, or that O is the void and formless infinite from which the secondary and primary qualities composing the entities are acquired.

Now something new is being introduced. Although the "conquest" of entities extracted from the void and formless infinite belongs to the K link, that is, it is the result of a knowledge activity, supposing that O already contains undeveloped potentialities leads Bion to propose the thesis that the development of these potentialities is also already part of becoming O, of transformation in O. If O already comprises a certain "evolutionary" direction, the impact of O corresponds to *being "become" by O*, letting oneself be done by O.

Between the two meanings of O (referred to in (i) and (ii) from the excerpt above) there is – without this being very clear in the text – a curious relationship. Being become by O seems to imply a "constructive" movement in which O imposes itself with its "development" potential. Becoming O, understood now as a void and formless infinite, is, on the contrary, a deconstructive movement back to baseless, to the dark nights of the soul. In the first case it is *letting oneself be done by O*, in the other is *letting oneself be undone in O*.

In both cases, something that goes beyond K link is at stake; in both cases it is an experience of the unconscious that is perfectly recognizable by the psychoanalyst. Neither of the meanings of O and the impact of O, or – seen from the other side – of the surrender to O, can be abolished. However, it is undeniable that these two meanings of O are as necessary as they are incompatible (leaving aside the most problematic: the Platonizing one). We approach the most fundamental notion: that of undecidability as far as our notions of O are concerned.

Returning to the problem of resistance, Bion will say that it is directed against the transformations of O into K which, in a way, are already part of the evolution of O's potentialities, and which thus threaten the individual with the transformation in O. It is to this extent that resistance can be expressed as an interruption in the process of knowing. This interruption not only prevents the transformation in O and the steps of a transformation in K which would already be excessively close to the transformation in O, and therefore threatening, but it also institutes an unlimited permanence in K. Knowledge is fought in its efficiency of conducting to transformation in O, using knowledge itself in this combat. Bion's example is the preference to see a photo, a reproduction of a work of art, instead of exposure to the work of art itself. Even before a work of art, this contact can be avoided if we put ourselves in the position of the person who observes the fact (at least when it comes to a painting or figurative sculpture) that it is only the reproduction of a landscape or of a human figure. Resistance is always resistance to contact with the experience of the thing – enhanced when it is a work of art – without the mediation of representations, transformations in K, L or H. The contact with the thing or work of art would be precisely the exposure to O as a potentiality, letting oneself be done by O. However, letting oneself be done by O is indissolubly linked with letting oneself be undone in O. In aesthetic experience, the two meanings of O, despite their antagonism, are requested, albeit in different degrees, according to the work and the relationship that each one manages to establish with it.

In the experience of the unconscious implied in psychoanalysis, it is necessary, in the same way, to recognize both the dimension of becoming and of undoing. Nothing intrinsic to a given interpretation assures us that it will be able to pass through this narrow, but two-way track, of "letting oneself be done by" and "undoing in". It can always become an obstacle or be ineffective.

> Any interpretation may be accepted in K but rejected in O; acceptance in O means that acceptance of an interpretation enabling the patient to know that part of himself to which attention has been drawn is felt to involve 'being' or 'becoming' that person.
>
> (Bion [1965] 2014, p. 273)

The resistance is always located in the transit from K to O; it is this that must be interdicted, even if, at times, the interruption must occur earlier, that is, between links of K that already threaten with the transition to O. Continuing:

> For many interpretations this price is paid. But some are felt to involve too high a price, notably those which the patient regards as involving him in 'going mad' or committing murder of himself or someone else, or becoming 'responsible' and therefore guilty. There is one class of interpretations, which seems to illuminate good qualities, but objection to which is not so easy to understand. The extreme example – interpretations which involve 'becoming O' – are dreaded as inseparable from megalomania, or what psychiatrists or the public might name delusions of grandeur or other diagnoses implying grave pathological disorder.
>
> (Bion [1965] 2014, p. 273)

The most interesting thing in this comment about resistance, in our view, is the fact that resistance is linked to the notion of "price". Becoming O (by letting oneself be done by it or being undone in it) carries a cost. Some costs are easier to pay than others. Among the difficult ones, however, there are costs that are high because they impose the experience of a limit – responsibility and guilt –there are also high costs that correspond to the risk of an experience of the unlimited – delusions of grandeur, megalomania, madness. Undoing in O, effectively breaks, as in the case of certain very strong aesthetic experiences, the frames of individual and group mind. It may also be "necessary" to resist, as is the case of patients who report the unbearability of situations of exaltation (for example, receiving a compliment, even if deserved, or exercising a competence fully and successfully). For some patients it seems impossible to rediscover the limits in the field of the unlimited, so they feel they can go astray in a megalomaniac drift, in a manic outbreak etc. We believe that there are patients who need to remain markedly depressed and/or inhibited in order to defend themselves from experiences of undoing in O (becoming O) in which prevail the disconnected energies, the pure quantities, to use Freudian language.

Let us skip over a few paragraphs to continue our research on the status of O, and on the resistance to the imminent transition to O. In dealing with the patient, the analyst

> ... cannot 'win' it 'from the void and formless infinite' of the analysand's personality, but only from the elements of the statement that the analysand has won from his own 'void and formless infinite'.
>
> (Bion [1965] 2014, p. 276)

We work on transformations of transformations of O; perhaps, at best, about the "emerging world of murky and deep waters", never on the void and formless infinite of the patient.

> Nothing is to be gained from telling the patient what he already knows unless what he 'knows' is being used to exclude what he 'is' (K opposed to O).
>
> (Bion [1965] 2014, p. 276)

Mirroring, the mere repetition, does not produce any circular movement, although a very sophisticated explanatory interpretation is capable of generating a drift without return. The good interpretation – the one that establishes an orbit and circulates through an adequate diameter – will be the one that allows the fulfilment of a circuit that leads from O to O, through the sequence of transformations that originate in patient's O; conquests initiated by the patient himself in his statements and free associations. These processes must be leveraged by the analyst's interpretations, so that they can return to O, that is, provide the patient with an "experience of the unconscious".

This cycle requires O to be, at the same time, the void and formless infinite – which justifies, to a certain extent, its translation by Zero – from which the figures are acquired and, also, a field of possibilities not yet developed, but which may be so, through the sequences of transformations, until the cycle of return to O can be concluded.

What can happen is that the passage through these various moments of the cycle and, mainly, the threat of returning to O (or Zero) generates resistance not only in the analysand, but also in the analyst. In this situation, interpretations can be articulated and given, carrying the (disguised) function of interrupting the circuit and avoiding the experience of turbulence in the analyst's mind. The more emphatic the analysand's communication, the more he uses projective identifications, the more hyperbolic elements are present, and the greater the analyst's tendency to resort to interpretations related to column 2. Let us return to the text:

> Any statement may be supposed to include dimensions represented by every grid category. Not all dimensions have evolved (or been won) from

the formlessness in which the potentiality for all distinctions exists. Therefore a statement can lack a varying number of classifiable dimensions because they remain undifferentiated potentialities. Epistemologically a statement may be regarded as evolved when any dimension can have a grid category assigned to it. For purposes of interpretation the statement is insufficiently evolved until its column 2 dimension is apparent. When the column 2 dimension has evolved, the statement can be said to be ripe for interpretation; its development as material for interpretation has reached maturity.

(Bion [1965] 2014, p. 276)

In this excerpt Bion emphasizes the assumption of O as an inaccessible field of potential. The analysand's transformations of O – interconnected to the analyst's transformations – are fundamentally ways of developing those potentialities. They are also ways of filling and giving form to the void and formless infinite, as long as it is understood, at this moment, that the forms acquired to the void would be as if prefigured by the field of potentialities. O, here, is Origin. However, among the inevitable potentialities of this process, on which the analyst must necessarily rely, it concerns the emergence of column 2 elements, that is, speeches that have the function of: filling, interrupting, evacuating, etc. The emergence of resistances is, therefore, contained in that field of O's undeveloped potentialities. But what would be the reason for resistances, if O were only the Origin to be fully developed in life processes? What is the threat of becoming O in this case? It is here that the notion of the void and formless infinite is imposed from where murky and deep waters emerge. This is the dreaded transition: the transition to Zero, to the void and formless infinite. This is the "origin" of the resistance. Let us continue:

In terms of analytic theory it is approximately correct, but only approximately, to say that the conditions for an interpretation have arrived when the patient's statements provide evidence that resistance is operating: the conditions are complete when the analyst feels aware of resistance in himself – not counter-transference which must be dealt with by analysis of the analyst, but resistance to the reaction he anticipates from the analysand if he gives the interpretation.

(Bion [1965] 2014, p. 277)

While the patient's transformations – with some participation of the analyst – are evolving, an interpretation is precocious and, if given at this moment, will probably attest only to the analyst's difficulty in maintaining ignorance and impotence. Interpretation becomes necessary when column 2 elements begin to emerge, first on the patient, but then on himself, in the form of an attempt to avoid certain reactions on the patient. The analyst feels that he loses his freedom for fear of triggering very strong resistance reactions in the patient. He tends to protect himself by becoming silent or saying something that is in itself of the order of a column 2 element. This would be the appropriate moment for the interpretation in which a resistance is faced with a double risk: for the patient, the risk of transformation in O; for the analyst, the risk of confronting the turbulences the analysand can cause. And in continuity of the text:

> So far the 'distance' between the analysand's statement (association) and the analyst's statement (interpretation) has been stated in terms of time required for the emergence of the column 2 element in the statement of the analysand and 'proto-resistance', to coin a phrase, in the analyst to a response that has not yet been made.
>
> (Bion [1965] 2014, p. 277)

The term proto-resistance appears first as an attempt by the analyst to interrupt the transformation processes and, ultimately, the transformation into O, to protect the patient and himself from exposure to O, whether in the sense of being done by O, or in the sense of undoing in O. But "the analyst's proto-resistance must be projection of his own resistance to one dimension of his proposed interpretation" (Bion [1965] 2014, p. 277). It is, therefore, the analyst's resistance to a dimension of his own interpretation. When this proto-resistance operates in a dominant way,

> The interpretation he does give is a theory, known to be false, *vis-à-vis* an unknown contingent circumstance, but maintained as a barrier against turbulence expected to occur were it not so maintained ...
>
> (Bion [1965] 2014, p. 277)

On the whole, considering the antagonistic and complementary meanings of O – on the one hand, undeveloped potentialities, but crying out for development, that is, *Origin* and, on the other, void and formless infinite, that is, the nothingness of entities, the baseless, *Zero* – at the same time, it is necessary to think of both O in its imminence and O in its resistance, in such a way that one cannot be conceived without the other. The same forces that generate all transformation processes place barriers to these processes. These forces are what Bion finally names, on the last page of the book, it is the unconscious:

> Confronted with the unknown, "the void and formless infinite", the personality of whatever age fills the void (saturates the element), provides a form (names and binds a constant conjunction) and gives boundaries to the infinite (number and position). Pascal's phrase, "*Le silence éternel de ces espaces infinis m'effraie*" can serve as an expression of intolerance and fear of the 'unknowable' and hence of the unconscious in the sense of the undiscovered or the unevolved.
>
> (Bion [1965] 2014, p. 279)

What remains to be said is that this intolerance to the unconscious is already contained within itself as one of the undeveloped and lasting potentialities of this same field and, therefore, the experience of the unconscious, which is proper to psychoanalysis, necessarily includes all these movements and their own obstacles.

Reference

Bion, W.R. ([1965] 2014). Transformations. In: *The Complete Works of W.R. Bion, Vol. V*, ed. C. Mawson. London: Karnac Books, pp. 115–280.

References

Bion, W.R. (1959). Attacks on Linking. *The International Journal of Psychoanalysis*, 40: 308–315.

Bion, W.R. ([1962] 2014). Learning from Experience. In: *The Complete Works of W.R. Bion, Vol. IV*, ed. C. Mawson. London: Karnac Books, pp. 247–365.

Bion, W.R. ([1963] 2014). Elements of Psycho-Analysis. In: *The Complete Works of W. R. Bion, Vol. V*, ed. C. Mawson. London: Karnac Books, pp. 1–86.

Bion, W.R. ([1965] 2014). Transformations. In: *The Complete Works of W.R. Bion, Vol. V*, ed. C. Mawson. London: Karnac Books, pp. 115–280.

Bion, Wilfred R. ([1965] 2014). Memory and Desire. In: *The Complete Works of W.R. Bion, Vol. VI*, ed. C. Mawson. London: Karnac Books.

Bion, Wilfred R. ([1967] 2014). Notes on Memory and Desire. In: *The Complete Works of W.R. Bion, Vol. VI*, ed. C. Mawson. London: Karnac Books.

Bion, W.R. ([1967] 2014). Second Thoughts: Selected Papers on Psychoanalysis. In: *The Complete Works of W.R. Bion, Vol. VI*, ed. C. Mawson. London: Karnac Books.

Bion, Wilfred R. ([1970] 2014). Attention and Interpretation: A Scientific Approach to Insight in Psycho-Analysis and Groups. In: *The Complete Works of W.R. Bion, Vol. VI*, ed. C. Mawson. London: Karnac Books.

Bion, W.R. ([1992] 2014). Cogitations. In: *The Complete Works of W.R. Bion, Vol. XI*, ed. C. Mawson. London: Karnac Books, pp. 1–350.

Bléandonu, G. (1993). *Wilfred R. Bion. A vida e a obra 1897–1979* [*Wilfred R. Bion: Life and Work, 1897–1979*], trans. L.L. Hoory and M. Mortara. Rio de Janeiro: Imago Editora.

Cintra, E.U. and Ribeiro, M.F.R. (2018). *Por que Klein?* [*Why Klein?*]. São Paulo: Escuta.

Eco, U. (1989). *The Open Work*. Cambridge, MA: Harvard University Press.

Fairbairn, W.R.D. ([1952] 1981). *Psychoanalytic Studies of the Personality*. London: Routledge & Kegan Paul.

Figueiredo, L.C. (1999). *Palavras cruzadas entre Freud e Ferenczi* [*Crosswords between Freud and Ferenczi*]. São Paulo: Escuta.

Figueiredo, L.C. (2003). Verleugnung. A desautorização do processo perceptivo [Verleugnung: The disauthorization of the perceptual process]. In: *Elementos para a clínica contemporânea* [*Elements for the Contemporary Clinic*]. São Paulo: Escuta.

Figueiredo, L.C. (2003a). A clínica borderline [The borderline clinic]. In: *Elementos para a clínica contemporânea* [*Elements for the Contemporary Clinic*]. São Paulo: Escuta.

Figueiredo, L.C. (2008). Presença, Implicação e Reserva [Presence, Implication and Reservation]. In: L.C. Figueiredo and N. Coelho Jr., *Ética e Técnica em Psicanálise* [*Ethics and Technique in Psychoanalysis*], 2nd expanded edition. São Paulo: Escuta.

Figueiredo, L.C., Tamburrino, G. and Ribeiro, M. (2011). *Bion em nove lições. Lendo Transformações* [*Bion in Nine Lessons: Reading Transformations*]. São Paulo: Editora Escuta.

Freud, S. (1911). Formulations on the Two Principles of Mental Functioning. In: *The Standard Edition of the Complete Psychological Works of Sigmund Freud, Vol. XII, (1911–1913)*, trans. J. Strachey. London: The Hogarth Press and the Institute of Psychoanalysis, pp. 218–226.

Freud, S. (1920). Beyond the Pleasure Principle. In: *The Standard Edition of the Complete Psychological Works of Sigmund Freud, Vol. XVIII, (1920–1922)*, trans. J. Strachey. London: The Hogarth Press and the Institute of Psychoanalysis, pp. 7–64.

Freud, S. ([1932] 1933). Lecture XXI: The Dissection of the Psychical Personality. New Introductory Lectures on Psycho-Analysis. In: *The Standard Edition of the Complete Psychological Works of Sigmund Freud, Vol. XXII, (1932–1936)*, trans. J. Strachey. London: The Hogarth Press and the Institute of Psychoanalysis.

Frochtengarten, J. (2012). Book review of Bion em nove lições: lendo *Transformações* [Bion in Nine Lessons: Reading Transformations]. *Revista Brasileira de Psicanálise*, 46(3): 229–232. Available at: http://pepsic.bvsalud.org/scielo.php?script=sci_a rttext&pid=S0486-641X2012000300016 [accessed 25 May 2024].

Gerber, I. and Figueiredo, L.C. (2018). *Por que Bion?* [*Why Bion?*]. São Paulo: Zagodoni Editora.

Grotstein, J. (2007). *A Beam of Intense Darkness: Wilfred Bion's Legacy to Psychoanalysis.* London: Karnac Books.

Nehamas, A. (1985). *Nietzsche: Life as Literature.* Cambridge, MA and London: Harvard University Press.

Rocha Barros, E.M. da and E.L. da Rocha Barros (2011). Reflections on the Clinical Implications of Symbols. *International Journal of Psychoanalysis*, 92(4): 879–901.

Rocha Barros, E.M. da and E.L. da Rocha Barros (2016). The Function of Evocation in the Working Through of the Countertransference: Projective Identification, Reverie and the Expressive Function of the Mind-Reflection Inspired by Bion's Work. In: H. Levine and G. Civitarese (eds), *The W.R. Bion Tradition.* London: Routledge, pp. 141–154.

Symington, J. and Symington, N. (1999). *O pensamento clínico de Wilfred Bion* [*The Clinical Thought of Wilfred Bion*]. Lisbon: Climepsi.

Vermote, R. (2019). *Reading Bion.* New York and London: Routledge.

Zimerman, D. (2004). *Bion da Teoria à Prática. Uma leitura didática* [*Bion from Theory to Practice: A Didactic Reading*]. Porto Alegre: Artmed.

Index

absolute facts, 44
absolute reality, inaccessibility, 77
abstract categories, signs, 35
abstraction, unsaturated representation, 41
achievement, process, 76
acting out, 60
acting-outs, 28
action, understanding, 34
adequate diameter, notion, 84
aesthetic experience, presence, 13
affection, scatter, 54–55
affective-emotional experience, communication, 57
affective ideograms, 13
affective intensities, 29
affects: presentations, 59–60; somatic dimension, characterization, 29
α elements, production, 48
α-function: confusion, 48; operation, sense impressions, 48
α function, encompassing, 9
analysand: communication, 95; personality, 95; statement (association), analyst statement (interpretation) difference, 97; statement, matching, 84, 85
analysis: breakdown, occurrence, 27; manifested demand, 11; premonitions, relationship, 51; transformation, 52; transformation, colloquial sense (danger), 52
analyst: chronic murder, 53–54; experience, 67; interpretations, giving, 25, 96; judgement, 60; listening/self-listening, 3–4; material, direct evidence, 25; personality, aspects, 54; questions, asking, 44; relationship, wholeness/coherence, 45;

rivalry/envy/thieving propensities, impact, 68; statement (interpretation), analysand statement (association) difference, 97; statement, matching, 85; statements, emotional experience representation, 59
analytical action, modes, 52
analytic experience, 25; knowing/being, presence, 84–85
analytic intuition, favoring, 12
analytic theory, 96
analytic treatment, discoveries, 43
analyzing, experience, 24
Andreas-Salomé, Lou, 7
annotations, basis, 17
anxieties, intuition, 7
arrest, process, 87
arrogance, 19
artist, analogy, 26
assumption of form, 46
at-one-ment, writing form, 20
attacks on linking, 49
Attention and Interpretation (Bion), 3, 13
awareness, development/growth, 51

becoming, 20, 92, 94; movement, 80
becoming O: absence, 84; involvement, 94; transition, 85
becoming, process, 83
becoming what one is, 20–21
being, 59, 94; presence, 84–85
being at one with, 20
being O, 92
Berkeley, George, 87
β-elements, 38
β elements: impact, 61–62; transformation, 28
Beyond the Pleasure Principle (Freud), 45